Hepatitis C and B: Management and Treatment

Second Edition

Thierry Poynard MD, PhD

Professor of Hepatology and Gastroenterology,
Head Department Hépato-Gastroenterology,
Groupe Hospitalier Pitié-Salpêtrière, University Paris 6,
and Assistant Director Research Laboratory
Liver Physio-Pathology
CNRS FRE 2443 Paris

TOURO COLLEGE LIBRARY
Main Campus Midtown

WITHDRAWN

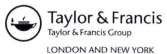

Taylor & Francis
Taylor & Francis Group

LONDON AND NEW YORK

A MARTIN DUNITZ BOOK

MT

First published in the United Kingdom in 2004
by Taylor and Francis, an imprint of the Taylor and Francis Group,
2 Park Square, Milton Park, Abingdon, Oxfordshire OX14 4RN

Tel.:   +44 (0) 1235 828600
Fax.:   +44 (0) 1235 829000
E-mail: info@dunitz.co.uk
Website: http://www.dunitz.co.uk

A CIP record for this book is available from the British Library.

Data available on application

ISBN 1-84184-369-5

Distributed in North and South America by

Taylor & Francis
2000 NW Corporate Blvd
Boca Raton, FL 33431, USA

Within Continental USA
Tel.: 800 272 7737; Fax.: 800 374 3401
Outside Continental USA
Tel.:   561 994 0555; Fax.: 561 361 6018
E.mail: orders @crcpress.com

Distributed in the rest of the world by
Thomson Publishing Services
Cheriton House
North Way
Andover, Hampshire SP10 5BE, UK
Tel: +44 (0) 1264 332424
E-mail: salesorder.tandf@thomsonpublishingservices.co.uk

Composition by Wearset Ltd, Boldon, Tyne and Wear
Printed and bound in Great Britain by The Cromwell Press Ltd

2/17/05

Contents

Introduction

This book aims to present a contemporary approach to the natural history and to the management of chronic hepatitis C and B virus infections.

Chronic hepatitis C virus infection is a major cause of chronic liver disease, with increasing mortality throughout the world. However, there is now very effective treatment that enables a physician to eradicate the virus in 60% of cases and to reduce the progression to cirrhosis in the remainder; even cases of cirrhosis reversal are now observed. This infection should therefore be detected and treated as necessary.

Chronic hepatitis B virus infection is still a major cause of chronic liver disease and of mortality throughout the world, despite the efficacy of the vaccine. However, its natural history is now better understood, with a better knowledge of mutations and a spectacular increase in the sensitivity of viral load assessment. In recent years the treatment has also been improved by the approval of lamivudine and adefovir: these nucleosides have very rapid efficacy in comparison to interferon and are better tolerated.

Finally, liver biopsy used to be considered an essential procedure in order to reach rational decisions in patients with chronic hepatitis C and B. However, limitations of liver biopsy are now better known: in particular, there can be a huge sampling error for staging fibrosis and grading necrosis. Non-invasive biochemical markers have been recently improved and could be used as an alternative to liver biopsy. To conclude this text, therefore, a dedicated chapter updates the advantages and limits of histological and biochemical markers of liver injury in chronic viral hepatitis C and B.

Thierry Poynard MD, PhD
Paris 2004

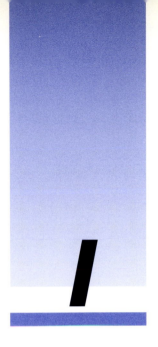

Hepatitis C

Natural history of hepatitis C: Epidemiology

It took many years before communities realized the importance of the hepatitis C epidemic (Figure 1.1). Chronic hepatitis C virus (HCV) infection is estimated to affect 170 million individuals worldwide[1] (Figure 1.2). These individuals are at risk of developing hepatologic and nonhepatologic manifestations.

Hepatitis C can cause cirrhosis, digestive hemorrhage, liver failure and liver cancer. Together with alcoholic cirrhosis, hepatitis C is the major reason for liver transplants in Europe and in the United States. Cumulative evidence strongly suggests that the increase of mortality due to hepatocellular carcinoma in most Western countries is due to hepatitis C infection[2-5] (Figure 1.3).

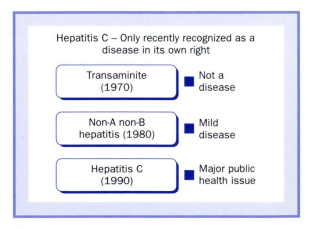

Figure 1.1
Perception of HCV epidemic.

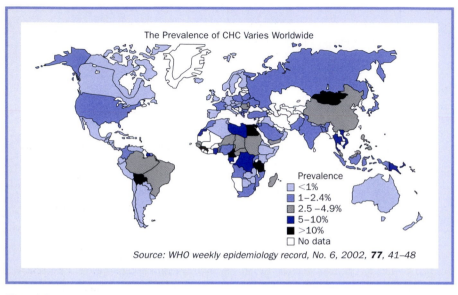

Figure 1.2
World prevalence of HCV.

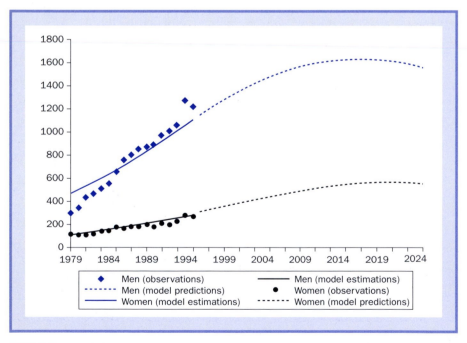

Figure 1.3
Increase in mortality related to primary liver cancer due to hepatitis C in France. Adapted with permission.[4]

Table 1.1 Risk groups for HCV infection.

Major high-risk groups	*Blood transfusion before 1991.*
	Frequent exposure to blood products: hemophilia, transplants, hemodialysis, chronic renal failure, gamma globulins, cancer chemotherapy.
	Injection drug use even briefly many years ago.
	Health-care workers with needle-stick accidents.
	Infants born to HCV-infected mothers, particularly those coinfected with HIV.
Moderate-risk groups	*High-risk sexual behavior, multiple partners, history of herpes simplex 2 infection.*
	Cocaine use, with sharing of intranasal administration equipment.

Transmission of HCV is mainly related to contact with blood and blood products (Table 1.1). Blood transfusions and the use of shared, nonsterilized needles and syringes have been the main causes of the spread of HCV. With routine blood screening for HCV antibody (1991 in most countries), transfusion-related hepatitis C has virtually disappeared. At present, injection drug use is the most common risk factor. However, many other patients acquire HCV without any known exposure to blood or to drug injection. A recent survey suggests that patients with high-risk sexual behavior are at higher risk, perhaps in association with herpes simplex 2 infection.[6]

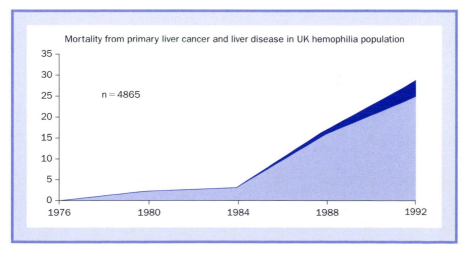

Figure 1.4
Increase in mortality related to primary liver cancer and liver disease in UK hemophilia population. Adapted with permission.[2]

Natural history of hepatitis C: Hepatic manifestations

2

The major hepatologic consequence of hepatitis C is the progression to cirrhosis and its potential complications: hemorrhage, hepatic insufficiency and primary liver cancer.

Current understanding of HCV infection has been advanced by the concept of liver fibrosis progression[7,8] (Figures 2.1 and 2.2). Fibrosis is the deleterious but variable consequence of chronic inflammation. It is characterized by the deposition of an extracellular matrix component, leading to the distortion of the hepatic architecture with impairment of liver microcirculation and liver cell functions. Usually, HCV is lethal only when it leads to cirrhosis, the last stage of liver fibrosis. Therefore, an estimate of fibrosis progression represents an important surrogate endpoint for evaluation of the vulnerability of an individual patient and for assessment of the impact of treatment on natural history.

Fibrosis stages and necroinflammatory activity grades

Activity and fibrosis are two major histologic features of chronic hepatitis C which are included in the different proposed classifications.[9–12] One of the few validated scoring systems is the METAVIR system.[11,12] This system assesses histologic lesions in chronic hepatitis C by two separate scores, one for necroinflammatory grade (A for activity) and another for the stage of fibrosis (F). These scores were defined as follows. Stages of fibrosis (F) (Figure 2.1): F0 = no fibrosis, F1 = portal fibrosis without septa, F2 = portal

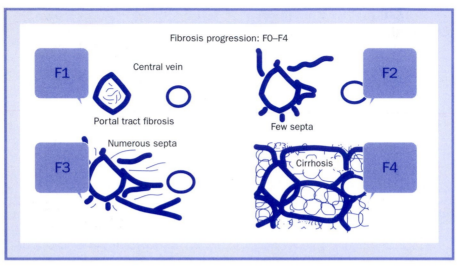

Figure 2.1
The METAVIR fibrosis staging system. F0 is normal liver (no fibrosis). F1 = portal fibrosis; F2 = few septa; F3 = many septa; F4 = cirrhosis.

fibrosis with rare septa, F3 = numerous septa without cirrhosis, F4 = cirrhosis. Grade for activity (A): A0 = no histologic activity, A1 = minimal activity, A2 = moderate activity, A3 = severe activity. The degree of activity was assessed by integration of the severity of the intensity of both piecemeal (periportal) necrosis and lobular necrosis, as described in a simple algorithm.[12] The intra- and interobserver variations of this METAVIR scoring system are lower than those of the widely used Knodell scoring system.[9,10] For METAVIR fibrosis stages, there is an almost perfect concordance (kappa = 0.80) among pathologists. The Knodell scoring system has a nonlinear scale. There is no stage 2 for fibrosis (range 0–4), and the activity grade ranges from 0 to 18 with the sum of periportal necrosis, intralobular and portal inflammation grades. The modified Histologic Activity Index is

more detailed with four different features and continuous grades, and the modified fibrosis staging includes six stages.

Activity grade, which represents the necrosis feature, is not a good predictor of fibrosis progression.[7] In fact, fibrosis alone is the best marker of ongoing fibrogenesis.[13,14] Fibrosis stage and inflammatory grade are correlated, but for one-third of patients, there is a discordance. Clinicians should not take a "significant activity" as a surrogate marker of "a severe disease". The clinical hallmarks of major necrosis and inflammation, that is, severe acute hepatitis and fulminant hepatitis, are finally very rare in comparison to hepatitis B. Even in immunologically compromised patients, there are very few acute flare-ups in patients with chronic hepatitis C.

The dynamic view of fibrosis progression

The fibrosis stage summarizes the vulnerability of a patient and is predictive of the progression to cirrhosis[7] (Figure 2.2). There is a strong correlation for fibrosis stages, almost linear, with age at biopsy and duration of infection. This correlation was not observed between activity grades.

Because of the informative value of fibrosis stage, there is an interest for clinicians to assess the speed of the fibrosis progression. The distribution of fibrosis progression rates suggests the presence of at least three populations: one population of "rapid fibrosers", a population of "intermediate fibrosers" and one population of "slow fibrosers" (Figure 2.3). Therefore, the expression of a mean (or median) fibrosis progression rate per year (stage at the first biopsy/duration of infection) and of a mean

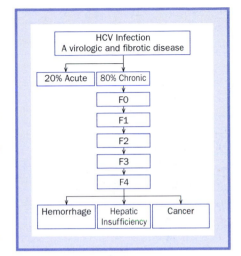

Figure 2.2
The model of fibrosis progression from infection to complications. Estimated key numbers of HCV natural history from literature and our database. The median time from infection (F0) to cirrhosis (F4) is 30 years. The mortality rate at 10 years for cirrhosis is 50%. The transition probability per year from noncomplicated cirrhosis to each of the complications is around 3%.

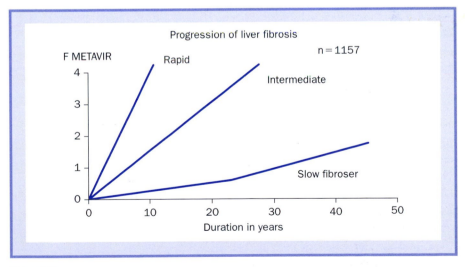

Figure 2.3
Progression of liver fibrosis in patients with chronic hepatitis C. By the median fibrosis progression rate, in untreated patients, the median expected time to cirrhosis is 30 years (intermediate fibroser). 33% of patients have an expected median time to cirrhosis of less than 20 years (rapid fibroser); 31% will progress to cirrhosis in more than 50 years, if ever (slow fibroser). Adapted with permission.[7]

expected time to cirrhosis does not signify that the progression to cirrhosis is universal and inevitable. By the median fibrosis progression rate, in untreated patients, the median expected time to cirrhosis is 30 years; 33% of patients have an expected median time to cirrhosis of less than 20 years, and 31% will progress to cirrhosis in more than 50 years, if ever (Figure 2.3).

The limitations of any estimate of fibrosis include (i) the difficulty in obtaining paired liver biopsies, (ii) the necessity for large numbers of patients to achieve statistical power and (iii) the sample variability in fibrosis distribution. Because the time elapsed between biopsies is relatively short (usually 12–24 months), the number of events (transition from one stage to another) is small. Therefore, the comparison between fibrosis progression rates requires a large sample size to observe significant differences. The slope of progression is difficult to assess because there is no large database with several biopsies. Therefore, the real slope is currently unknown, and even if there is a linear relationship between stages and age at biopsy or duration of infection, other models are

possible.[15] Recently, on a larger database, we confirmed that the fibrosis progression was mainly dependent on the age and the duration of infection, with four different periods with very slow, slow, intermediate and rapid slopes[16] (Figure 2.4).

Furthermore, liver biopsy has its own limit to assess liver fibrosis. Although it is the gold standard to score fibrosis, its value is limited by sample variability. See Chapter 3 for a discussion.

Factors associated with fibrosis progression

Factors associated and not associated with fibrosis are summarized in Table 2.1. Several factors have been shown to be associated with fibrosis progression rate:[4,7,16–20] duration of infection, age, male gender, consumption of alcohol, HIV coinfection, low CD4 count and necrosis grade. The progression from infection to cirrhosis depends strongly on sex and age[4,7] (Table 2.2). Metabolic conditions, such as overweight and diabetes, are emerging as independent cofactors of fibrogenesis.[21,22]

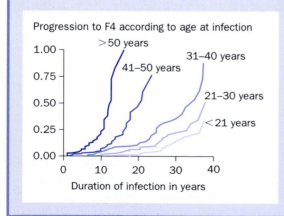

Figure 2.4
Probability of fibrosis progression to cirrhosis (F4) according to age at infection. Modeling in 2313 patients with known duration of infection. Adapted with permission.[16]

Table 2.1 Factors associated or not with fibrosis progression.

Associated in uni- and multivariate analysis	Not sure	Not associated
Fibrosis stage	Inflammation	Last serum viral load
Age at infection	Hemochromatosis heterozygote	Genotype non-3
Duration of infection	Cigarette consumption	Mode of infection
Age at biopsy	Moderate alcohol consumption	DR antigens
Consumption of alcohol	Genotype 3	Liver viral load
>50 g per day	Schistosomiasis	HCV-HVR1 complexity
HIV coinfection		
CD4 count <200/mL		
Female gender		
Necrosis		
Body-mass index and/or diabetes and/or steatosis		

Table 2.2 Multivariate analysis of risk factors by proportional hazards regression model for each fibrosis stage 20 years after HCV infection in 2313 patients. Adapted with permission.[16]

Risk factor	Stage F1		Stage F2		Stage F3		Stage F4	
	Relative hazard	P value	Relative hazard	P value	Relative hazard	P value	Relative hazard	P value
Infection after 30 years	4.4	<0.001	4.8	<0.001	11.5	<0.001	27.1	<0.001
Infection 21–30 years	2.3	<0.001	1.8	<0.001	2.5	<0.001	5.3	<0.001
Alcohol >50 g	1.3	0.20	3.0	<0.001	2.3	0.008	4.5	0.001
Male	1.0	0.76	1.3	0.03	1.9	<0.001	2.0	0.003
IV drug	1.6	<0.001	1.2	0.22	1.4	0.11	1.2	0.55
Activity A2, A3	0.8	0.009	1.2	0.21	2.0	<0.001	1.4	0.16

Age

The role of aging in fibrosis progression could be related to higher vulnerability to environmental factors, especially oxidative stress, and to reduction in blood flow, in mitochondria capacity, or in immune capacities.[23] The effect of age on fibrosis progression is so important that modeling the hepatitis C epidemic without taking into account the age of patients is not possible.

The estimated probability of progression per year for men aged between 61 and 70 years was 300 times greater than that for men aged between 21 and 40 years[4,16] (Figure 2.4).

Female gender

Female gender is associated with 10 times less rapid progression to cirrhosis than male whatever the age.[19] Estrogen modulates fibrogenesis in experimental injury, and blocks proliferation and fibrogenesis by stellate cells in primary culture. Estrogen could modify the expression of transforming growth factor and other soluble mediators.

Alcohol

The role of alcohol consumption has been established for daily doses greater than 40 or 50 g per day.[7,16–17] For lower doses, there are discordant results, even preliminary studies suggesting a protective effect of very small doses. Alcohol consumption is difficult to quantify, and conclusions must be prudent. However, it seems from these studies that the influence of alcohol is independent of other factors, is weaker than that of age, and is expected only at toxic levels of intake.

HIV coinfection

Several studies have demonstrated that patients coinfected with HCV and HIV have one of the most rapid fibrosis progression rates in comparison with monoinfected patients or

other liver diseases, even after taking into account age, sex and alcohol consumption[19,24–26] (Figure 2.5a). An HIV-infected patient with less than 200 CD4 cells/μL and drinking more than 50 g of alcohol daily has a median expected time to cirrhosis of 16 years, compared with 36 years for an HIV-infected patient with more than 200 CD4 cells/μL, and drinking 50 g or less of alcohol daily (Figure 2.5b).

Viral factors

Viral factors such as genotype, viral load at the time of the biopsy, and quasispecies are not associated with fibrosis.[7,27,28] Only genotype 3 is suspected, because of the steatosis associated with this genotype.[26] There are very few studies for the following factors, and more studies with high sample size are needed: fluctuations of HCV RNA, intrahepatic cytokine profiles, HLA class genotype, C282Y heterozygote hemochromatosis gene mutation, and cigarette consumption.

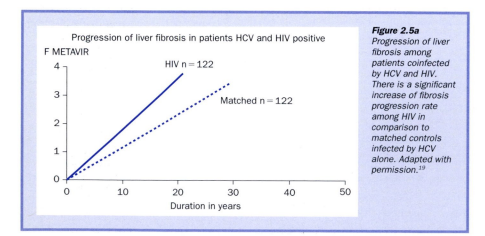

Figure 2.5a
Progression of liver fibrosis among patients coinfected by HCV and HIV. There is a significant increase of fibrosis progression rate among HIV in comparison to matched controls infected by HCV alone. Adapted with permission.[19]

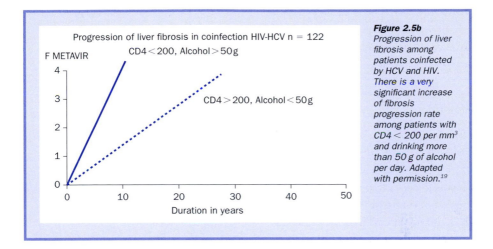

Figure 2.5b
Progression of liver fibrosis among patients coinfected by HCV and HIV. There is a very significant increase of fibrosis progression rate among patients with CD4 < 200 per mm³ and drinking more than 50 g of alcohol per day. Adapted with permission.[19]

Risk of fibrosis in patients with normal transaminases

Patients with repeated normal serum transaminase activity have a lower fibrosis progression rate than matched control patients with elevated transaminases[29,30] (Figure 2.6). However, there are still 15–19% of these patients with moderate or high fibrosis progression rates. Therefore, we recommend that the clinician assess the fibrosis stage, performing liver biopsy or biochemical markers in these PCR-positive patients. If the patient has septal fibrosis or portal fibrosis with a high fibrosis rate, treatment should be considered.

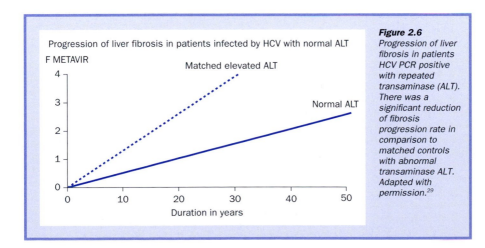

Figure 2.6
Progression of liver fibrosis in patients HCV PCR positive with repeated transaminase (ALT). There was a significant reduction of fibrosis progression rate in comparison to matched controls with abnormal transaminase ALT. Adapted with permission.[29]

Natural history of hepatitis C: Extrahepatic manifestations and quality of life

3

Numerous extrahepatic manifestations have been reported with hepatitis C virus (HCV) infection, including fatigue, mixed cryoglobulinemia, porphyria cutanea tarda, membranous glomerulonephritis, sicca syndrome, thyroiditis and high prevalence of autoantibodies.[31–35] We analyzed a cross-sectional study including 1614 patients.[31,34] Overall prevalence of the extrahepatic manifestations is shown in Table 3.1. By multivariate analysis, three main risk factors were associated with the presence of clinical or biological extrahepatic manifestations: advanced age, female sex and extensive liver fibrosis. There was no association with histologic activity grade.

Clinical manifestations

The extrahepatic clinical manifestations are particularly frequent, 74% of patients presenting at least one, with a preponderance of rheumatic (that is, arthralgia, myalgia and paresthesia) and cutaneomucous (pruritus, sicca syndrome and Raynaud's phenomenon) symptoms. Six manifestations had a prevalence above 10% including, in decreasing order, fatigue, arthralgia, paresthesia, myalgia, pruritus and sicca syndrome. This may reflect the nonspecific prevalence of these symptoms, as there is no control population matched for age and sex. Psychiatric disorders, especially depression and anxiety, and more frequent among HCV than non-HCV infected male controls.[33–35]

Systemic lupus erythematosus, Sjögren's syndrome, rheumatoid arthritis and dermatomyositis are uncommon in HCV-positive patients, suggesting a fortuitous association.

Table 3.1 Prevalence of clinical and biological extrahepatic manifestations in HCV-positive patients (decreasing order). Adapted with permission.[25]

	Percentage	95% CI
Clinical extrahepatic manifestation		
Tested in 1614 patients		
Fatigue	53	51–56
Arthralgia	23	21–26
Paresthesia	17	15–19
Myalgia	15	14–17
Pruritus	15	13–17
Sicca syndrome	11	10–13
Arterial hypertension	10	8–11
Diabetes	7	5–8
Raynaud's phenomenon	3.5	2.6–4.5
Abnormal thyroid function	3.4	2.0–4.0
Psoriasis	3	2–4
At least one clinical manifestation	74	72–77
Biological extrahepatic manifestation		
(Total tested)		
Cryoglobulin (1083)	40	37–43
Antinuclear Abs (874)	10	8–12
Low thyroxin (661)	10	8–13
Anti-smooth muscle Abs (873)	7	5–9
Anti-microsomal thyroid Abs (451)	5	3–8
Elevated creatininemia (1614)	3	2–4

The following extrahepatic manifestations were present in less than 2% of patients: purpura 1.5%, vasculitis 1%, lichen planus 1%, porphyria cutanea tarda 0.2%, antithyroglobulin Ab 2%, anti-liver-kidney microsomal Ab 2%, antimitochondrial Ab 1%, elevated thyroid-stimulating hormone 1%, low thyroid-stimulating hormone 1%, elevated thyroxin 1%. Ab = antibodies.

Systemic vasculitis, which is the severe symptomatic manifestation of cryoglobulinemia, although rare (1%), is the most frequent systemic inflammatory disease observed.

Due to the lymphotropism of HCV, a possible role of this viral agent has been suggested in the development of hemolymphopathies—in particular, B-cell non-Hodgkin's lymphoma in patients with HCV-mixed cryoglobulinemia.[36] Only one out of 1614 HCV patients of our cohort has developed non-Hodgkin's lymphoma to date.[32] Splenic lymphoma with villous lymphocytes is very rare but probably associated with HCV infection.[37]

Biological manifestations

Four biological abnormalities have a prevalence above 5%: cryoglobulin, antinuclear antibodies, anti-smooth muscle antibodies and low thyroxin level. At least one biological abnormality is present in 50% of patients.[31,32]

Mixed cryoglobulins is the predominant extrahepatic biological manifestation, identified in 40% of the 1083 patients we tested. All cryoglobulin-positive patients have mixed type II cryoglobulins (65%) or type III (35%). Five independent factors are significantly associated with the presence of a cryoglobulin: female sex, alcohol consumption above 50 g/day, HCV genotype 2 or 3, and extensive liver fibrosis. Cryoglobulin-positive patients present more arthralgia, arterial hypertension, purpura, and systemic vasculitis. However, considering the high frequency of positive cryoglobulin in HCV patients, severely symptomatic mixed cryoglobulinemia with vasculitis is rare, noted in 2–3% of cryoglobulin-positive patients.

Most systemic searches for biological extrahepatic manifestation in HCV-inffected patients revealed high prevalences of antinuclear (20–40%), anti-smooth muscle cell (20%), antithyroid (8–12%) and anticardiolipin (20%) antibodies. No association was observed between biological and clinical symptoms and autoantibodies positivity.

Numerous thyroid abnormalities have been observed among patients chronically infected by HCV, suggesting that HCV by itself or via an indirect immunologic pathway may induce thyroid dysfunction.[38] In our experience, clinically relevant thyroid abnormalities at the first visit—that is, before any interferon or other anti-HCV treatment—are rare. Low thyroxin levels are found in 10% of patients, but elevated thyroid stimulating hormone levels are noted in only 1%. Prevalences of antithyroid antibodies are in accordance with the age and sex ratio of the population studied.

Health-related quality of life

One way to assess the clinical impact of hepatic and extrahepatic manifestation among patients infected by HCV is to assess the health-related quality of life. Several studies have demonstrated that patients even without cirrhosis have an impaired quality of life[39–42] (Figure 3.1). The quality of life is impaired by the diagnosis itself but also by the virus in comparison to controls.

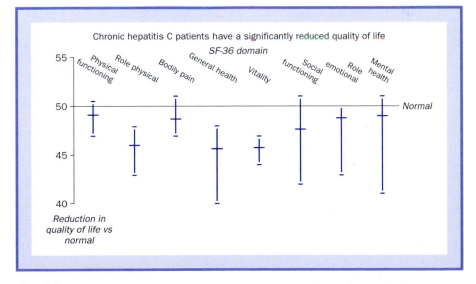

Figure 3.1
Quality of life is impaired among patients infected with hepatitis C.

Management protocols in chronic hepatitis C

4

There is no vaccine yet available; the prevention of hepatitis C lies in the minimalization of blood exposure. In the last 10 years, considerable progress has been made in the management of chronic hepatitis C, in terms of both achieving viral eradication and improving histology.[43]

Considering the natural history of hepatitis C, there are three different goals for treatment: (1) to prevent the occurrence of cirrhosis and its complications, (2) to reduce the extrahepatic manifestations, and (3) to prevent the contamination of other people (that is, surgeon or drug user). No treatment is needed in asymptomatic patients that are not at risk of progressing to cirrhosis or transmitting the virus. High alcohol consumption must be avoided and metabolic conditions (diabetes, overweight) improved.[44]

Worldwide approvals are not homogeneous across countries, and the aim of this chapter is to present the most up-to-date results. Since the first approval in 1990 (standard interferon regimen monotherapy with three injections three times a week TIW) to the approval in 2001 (combination of ribavirin and pegylated interferon [PEG-IFN]), several main regimens have been assessed in large trials: standard interferon alfa (alfa-2a or -2b, 3 MU TIW) for 24 weeks and then 48 weeks,[45] the combination of standard interferon (3 MU TIW) and ribavirin (1000 mg ribavirin if weight <75 kg, 1200 mg ≥ 75 kg) for 24 weeks or 48 weeks,[46–48] PEG-IFN 48 weeks (alfa-2a 180 μg, or alfa-2b at three doses: 0.5 μg, 1.0 μg, or 1.5 μg per kg),[49–51] and 48 weeks of combination PEG-IFN and ribavirin (different doses of PEG and ribavirin).[52–54] Combination therapy was always more effective than interferon monotherapy, even PEG-IFN monotherapy. The combination regimen in the first European approval was the combination of 1.5 μg PEG-IFN per kg and ribavirin adjusted on the weight as well (800 mg if weight <65 kg, 1000 mg between 65 and 85 kg and 1200 mg if weight >85 kg).

Summary of main progress

A summary of the main progress, of different approved regimens, on virologic endpoint (sustained virologic response) is shown in Figure 4.1. Results were presented according to HCV genotype, the main factor associated with viral response.

We have assessed the impact of 10 different regimens on both virologic endpoints and histologic endpoints in 3004 patients with paired biopsies[55,56] (Figure 4.2).

Efficacy of ribavirin and standard interferon combination regimen

Many lessons have been learned from the nonpegylated interferon and ribavirin that can be useful for the last approved combination with pegylated interferon (PEG-IFN).

Efficacy of combination regimen on viral endpoints

When the two pivotal trials of ribavirin and interferon combination were combined,[46–48] the database included 1744 treatment-naive patients. At the end of treatment, the percentage of patients with undetectable HCV RNA was significantly higher in the combination groups: 51% (260/505) in the IFN-R 48 week, 55% (278/505) in the IFN-R 24 week, 29% (147/503) in the IFN 48 week, and 29% in the IFN 24 week (66/231)

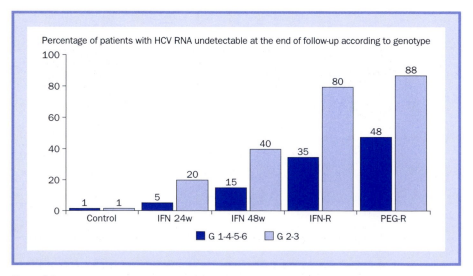

Figure 4.1
Progress in the treatment of chronic hepatitis C.

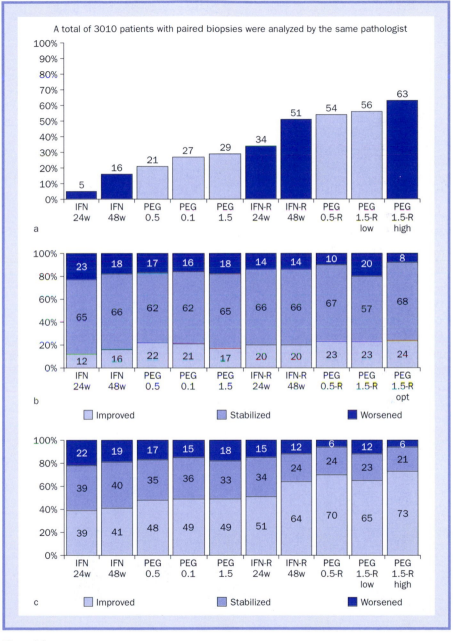

Figure 4.2
Virologic efficacy (panel a) of 10 different regimens (interferon and ribavirin) and impact on fibrosis stage (panel b) and necroinflammatory activity grade (panel c). Adapted with permission.[56]

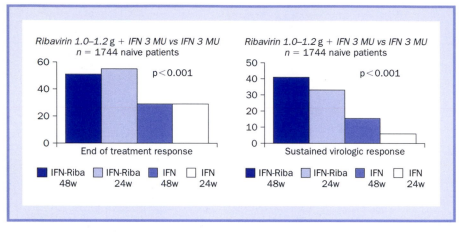

Figure 4.3
Efficacy of combination ribavirin-interferon at the end of the treatment (panel a) and at the end of 24 weeks' follow-up (panel b). Adapted with permission.[48]

(Figure 4.3a). At the end of the follow-up, the percentage of patients with sustained undetectable HCV RNA was also higher in the combination groups: 41% (205/505), 33% (166/505), 16% (82/503) and 6% (13/231), respectively, with significant differences between all these groups (Figure 4.3b).

These results demonstrated that there was a combination effect without duration effect on the end of treatment response, and that there was both a combination effect and a duration effect on the sustained response.

Even in virologic nonresponders, there was an improvement in transaminase (Figure 4.4a) activity and in mean serum viral load (Figure 4.4b) during treatment.

Efficacy of combination regimen on extrahepatic manifestations and on quality of life

Little is known concerning the efficacy of treatment on extrahepatic manifestations.

During the treatment and because of the adverse events, there was an impairment of health-related quality of life in combination to baseline value.[30–31] After the end of the treatment, there was an improvement of health-related quality of life in sustained responders in comparison to baseline level.[41,42] Studies describing the impact of treatment on the troublesome symptoms are sparse. In a study of 431 patients, a significant impact of antiviral therapy on fatigue and cryoglobulinemia after 18 months of follow-up was found[57] (Table 4.1). In severe symptomatic cryoglobulinemia, there was a clinical improvement by treatment. None of a wide range of other extrahepatic manifestations improved significantly in patients with a sustained response to treatment when compared with nonresponders, relapsers and untreated patients.[57]

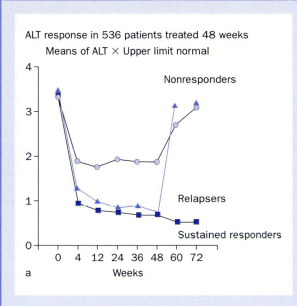

ALT response in 536 patients treated 48 weeks
Means of ALT × Upper limit normal

Nonresponders

Relapsers

Sustained responders

a   Weeks

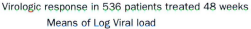

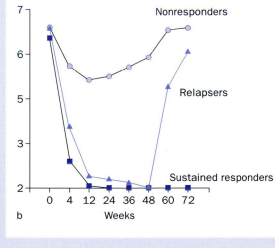

Virologic response in 536 patients treated 48 weeks
Means of Log Viral load

Nonresponders

Relapsers

Sustained responders

b   Weeks

Figure 4.4
Improvement of histology after combination ribavirin-interferon. Panel a Activity grade; panel b fibrosis progression rate. Adapted with permission.[48]

Table 4.1 Impact of antiviral treatment on clinical and biological extrahepatic manifestations in patients with chronic hepatitis C. Adapted with permission.[57]

Extrahepatic manifestations	Sustained responders	Others with persistently detectable HCV-RNA				p-value (Sustained responders vs all others)
		All others	Relapsers	Nonresponders	Untreated	
	n = 83	n = 348	n = 47	n = 225	n = 76	
Fatigue						
Baseline	58%	59%	55%	60%	61%	0.82
Month 18	31%	55%	60%	53%	55%	<0.001
Arthralgia						
Baseline	34%	30%	32%	31%	26%	0.53
Month 18	14%	14%	9%	15%	14%	0.93
Paresthesia						
Baseline	17%	17%	15%	19%	14%	0.94
Month 18	7%	9%	6%	8%	11%	0.67
Myalgia						
Baseline	19%	22%	23%	25%	13%	0.53
Month 18	8%	12%	9%	14%	9%	0.35
Sicca syndrome						
Baseline	10%	17%	21%	18%	13%	0.09
Month 18	2%	6%	11%	5%	5%	0.28
Diabetes						
Baseline	6%	5%	9%	5%	4%	0.84
Month 18	2%	3%	2%	4%	1%	0.99
Cryoglobulinemia						
Baseline	48%	45%	58%	44%	37%	0.69
Month 18	6% (2/34)	33% (38/115)				<0.001

Factors associated with treatment response and "a la carte" regimen

Careful analysis of pivotal trials has confirmed the independent prognostic values of five baseline characteristics.[46–48] HCV genotypes 2 and 3 were associated with better response to the combination than other genotypes. For viral load, the ROC curves showed that there was no threshold that had either a positive or negative predictive value. Therefore, the simplest way to classify viral load into high or low was to take the median, which was 3.5 million copies (now 800 000 IU/mL). For age, the threshold of 40 years seemed to have the best accuracy. Because the multivariate analysis showed that these five factors could explain only 20% of the variability of the sustained response, we need to identify the other independent factors.

Is treatment by interferon alone sufficient among patients with many favorable factors?

There is no place for interferon monotherapy at a dose of 3 million units three times a week for either 24 or 48 weeks even in the most favorable patient. Among patients with genotype 2 or 3 and low viral load, the sustained response rate was much greater with 24 weeks of combination regimen (71%) than with 48 weeks of interferon monotherapy (40% p < 0.001). Interferon monotherapy should be recommended only if combination interferon alfa-2b plus ribavirin therapy is contraindicated.

Duration of nonpegylated interferon and ribavirin combination regimen: 12, 24 or 48 weeks?

The first question was whether treatment can be stopped at 12 weeks in some subgroups because of a high probability of nonresponse. There was no consensus at an international conference.[58] From our data, this approach cannot be recommended because in the 48-week regimen, among the patients who had a positive PCR at 12 weeks, we observed a sustained response in 10% of patients. Even the 24-week regimen induces a sustained response in 4% of these patients. Furthermore, the antifibrotic effect of 24-week treatment in nonresponders is a benefit for patients.[55,56,59]

The choice of 24 or 48 weeks for nonpegylated interferon and ribavirin combination therapy has been clarified. The crucial time to make this decision is at 24 weeks based on the results of HCV PCR testing. In patients who are PCR negative at 24 weeks (59% of the patients in these studies), the goal is to reduce the relapse rate. There was an overall highly significant improvement with 48 weeks of treatment (74% sustained responders) versus 24 weeks (59% sustained responders). Since patients with many favorable response factors benefit less from 48 weeks of treatment, consideration can be given to stopping at 24 weeks in these patients. A simple strategy could be to consider only the HCV genotype, and stop treatment at week 24 in genotype 2 and 3 responders, since the sustained response was 82% in patients treated for 24 weeks versus 84% in patients treated for 48 weeks. However, from our results, it seems hazardous to recommend a strategy based only on virologic characteristics. There were in fact five independent response factors, and to take into account only one factor among these five is an oversimplification that could lead to errors in different populations or subgroups.[48] For example, we have determined that patients with genotype 2 or 3 who are PCR negative at 24 weeks and who have extensive fibrosis will have a better sustained response with 48 weeks of treatment, 80%, compared to 65% in patients whose treatment is stopped at 24 weeks. For a population of older men with extensive fibrosis, the choice of 48 weeks' duration in responders should not be based only on genotype and viral load.

Similarly, the recommendation of the international consensus conference[58] to treat patients with genotype 1 for only 6 months if the level of viremia is low was not correct, according to our results. This recommendation would lead to a reduction of 18% of the sustained response rate obtained by the 48-week regimen.

Table 4.2 Sustained virologic response to different regimens according to baseline characteristics.

Baseline characteristic	IFN-ribavirin 48 weeks	IFN-ribavirin 24 weeks
Genotype		
2 or 3	65%	67%
1, 4, 5 or 6	30%	18%
Mean HCV RNA		
$\leq 3.5 \times 10^6$ copies/mL	44%	40%
$> 3.5 \times 10^6$ copies/mL	38%	26%
Age		
≤ 40 years	48%	40%
> 40 years	34%	26%
Fibrosis stage		
No or portal fibrosis	43%	36%
Septal fibrosis or more	36%	23%
Gender		
Female	46%	39%
Male	38%	30%
Combination of virologic factors		
Genotype 2, 3 $\leq 3.5 \times 10^6$	65%	71%
Genotype 2, 3 $> 3.5 \times 10^6$	65%	62%
Genotype 1, 4, 5, 6 $\leq 3.5 \times 10^6$	33%	26%
Genotype 1, 4, 5, 6 $> 3.5 \times 10^6$	27%	10%
Combination of nonvirologic factors		
Women, ≤ 40 years, no of portal fibrosis	57%	56%
Men, > 40 years, septal fibrosis or more	34%	25%
Extreme favorable population		
Women, ≤ 40 years, no of portal fibrosis, genotype 2, 3 $\leq 3.5 \times 10^6$ cop	79%	69%
Extreme unfavorable population		
Men, > 40 years, septal fibrosis or more, genotype 1, 4, 5, 6 $> 3.5 \times 10^6$	9%	8%

Efficacy of PEG-IFN

Rational

Pegylation of proteins decreases clearance and thereby increases half-life and may extend biological activity. PEG-IFN, both alfa-2b and alfa-2a, has shown pharmacokinetic profiles allowing one injection per week (Figure 4.5).[60,61]

Efficacy of PEG-IFN in comparison with standard interferon

PEG-IFN alfa-2b (0.5, 1.0 and 1.5 µg per kg) has shown a greater efficacy than standard interferon regimen (3 MU TIW) on virologic endpoints, particularly at the end of treatment (Figure 4.6).[49] When genotype and

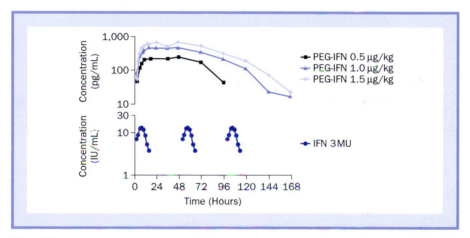

Figure 4.5
Pharmacokinetic single-dose profiles of PEG-IFN alfa-2b versus standard interferon alfa-2b (IFN 3 MU). Adapted with permission.[60]

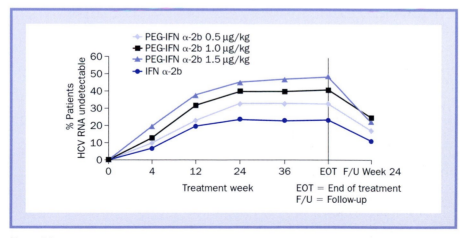

Figure 4.6
Efficacy of PEG-IFN alfa-2b: loss of HCV RNA over time. Adapted with permission.[49]

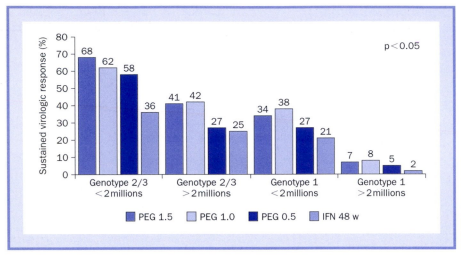

Figure 4.7
Efficacy of PEG-IFN alfa-2b monotherapy according to genotype and viral load. Adapted with permission.[49]

viral load were taken into account, the efficacy was low in genotype 1 and high viral load (Figure 4.7).

PEG-IFN alfa-2a (180 or 90 μg once a week) for 48 weeks has shown a greater

efficacy than standard interferon regimen (6 MU TIW alfa-2a for 12 weeks and then 3 MU TIW for the remaining 36 weeks of treatment)[50] (Figure 4.8).

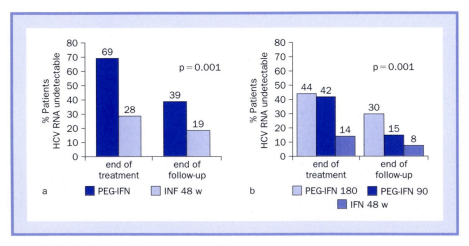

Figure 4.8
Efficacy of PEG-IFN alfa-2a monotherapy a: comparison of PEG 180 with standard interferon. Adapted with permission.[50] b: comparison of PEG 180 with PEG 90 and standard interferon in patients with bridging fibrosis or cirrhosis. Adapted with permission.[51]

Efficacy on extrahepatic manifestations and on quality of life

There were fewer adverse events in patients receiving lower doses of PEG-IFN alfa-2b than with standard interferon[49] (Figure 4.9).

Efficacy of combination of PEG-IFN alfa-2 and ribavirin

The combination of PEG-IFN with ribavirin is now the standard for first-line treatment of naive patients. Three large pivotal trials of PEG-IFN plus ribavirin combination therapy have been conducted.[52–55]

Efficacy on virologic endpoints

A randomized trial including 1530 patients has compared three regimens, two combinations of PEG-IFN alfa-2b and ribavirin and the standard interferon-ribavirin combination[52] (Figure 4.10). There was a significant difference in favor of PEG-IFN 1.5 μg per kg combination with ribavirin. This arm, in contrast to the other groups, had a fixed dose of ribavirin (800 mg), which was found retrospectively to be not optimized for patients with a weight of 65 kg or more (Figure 4.11). When the patients receiving the optimized dose (greater than 10.6 mg per kg; that is, more than 800 mg a day for a 75 kg person) were compared, there was a very significant difference in favor of PEG-IFN 1.5 μg versus the standard combination among patients infected with genotype 1 HCV, with an increase of sustained response from 33% to 48% (Figure 4.12). When patients with a good adherence were considered (at least 80% of the PEG-IFN and ribavirin dose during at least 80% of the 48 weeks), the percentage of sustained responder reached 63% among the genotype 1 (Figure 4.13).

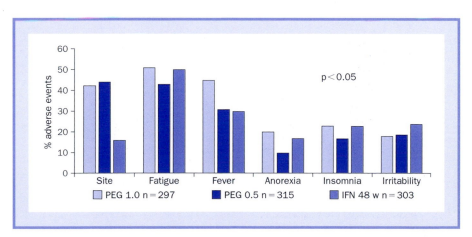

Figure 4.9
Adverse events in patients treated by PEG-IFN alfa-2b. There was significantly less anorexia, insomnia and irritability in patients receiving PEG 0.5 in comparison with standard interferon. Adapted with permission.[49]

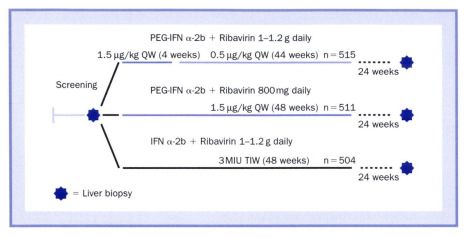

Figure 4.10
Study design of a randomized trial comparing the PEG-IFN ribavirin combination with the standard interferon ribavirin combination. Adapted with permission.[52]

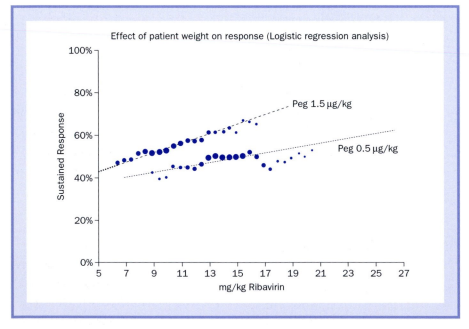

Figure 4.11
Effect of patient weight on sustained virologic response when treated by PEG-IFN alfa-2b and ribavirin. Adapted with permission.[52]

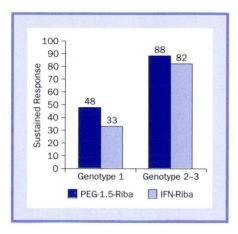

Figure 4.12
Efficacy of PEG-IFN and ribavirin optimized combination. Analysis adjusted for patients' weight. Adapted with permission.[52]

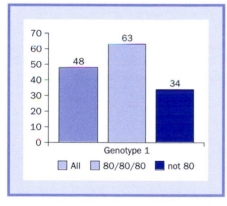

Figure 4.13
Efficacy in genotype 1 of PEG-IFN alfa-2b 1.5 μg and weight basis ribavirin. Analysis adjusted for patients' adherence. Adapted with permission.[63]

Factors associated with viral response

The same factors were associated with nonresponse and relapse[52] as for the standard combination:[48] HCV genotype 2 and 3, low HCV-RNA levels, body weight, age and degree of liver fibrosis. Therefore, post-approval studies must now establish one "a la carte" regimen for optimized combination.

In one study using PEG-IFN alfa-2a in combination with ribavirin for 24 or 48 weeks, patients with HCV-1 improved significantly their SVR when treated for longer, independently of pretreatment viral load, while no such difference was seen for patients with HCV-2 or HCV-3, again independently of pretreatment HCV-RNA levels. Furthermore, patients with HCV-1 responded better to higher dosages (1000–1200 mg/daily) or ribavirin.

On the basis of the results obtained in these trials, both forms of PEG-IFN have been approved in the United States and Europe for the treatment of chronic hepatitis C. The current recommendation is to use combination therapy with PEG-IFN and ribavirin as the new standard of treatment for all cases of chronic hepatitis C, except in situations where there are contraindications to ribavirin. The recommended dose of PEG-IFN alfa-2a is 180 μg/week, independently of body weight (Figures 4.14–4.16), while that of PEG-IFN alfa-2b is weight adjusted and fixed at 1.5 μg/kg per week with combination therapy and 1.0 μg/kg per week with monotherapy. The dose of ribavirin and the duration of therapy should be decided according to the HCV genotype. Patients with "easy-to-treat" HCV (HCV-2 and HCV-3) should be treated for 24 weeks while those with "difficult-to-treat" HCV (HCV-1 and, possibly, HCV-4) should be given a full dose of ribavirin (above 10.6 mg per kg) and treated for 48 weeks.

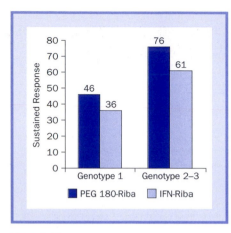

Figure 4.14
Efficacy of PEG-IFN alfa-2a 180 μg and ribavirin 1–1.2 g combination for 48 weeks. Adapted with permission.[53]

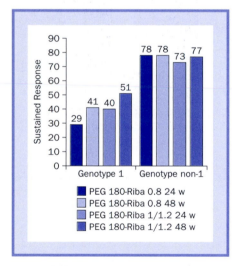

Figure 4.15
Efficacy of PEG-IFN alfa-2a 180 μg and ribavirin 1–1.2 g or 800 mg daily combination for 48 weeks or 24 weeks. Adapted with permission.[55]

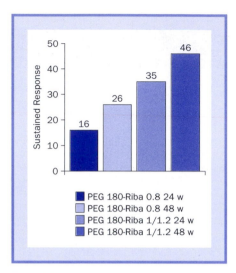

Figure 4.16
Efficacy of PEG-IFN alfa-2a 180 μg and ribavirin 1–1.2 g or 800 mg daily combination for 48 weeks or 24 weeks in genotype 1 with high viral load. Adapted with permission.[55]

Comparison between different PEG-IFNs in combination with Ribavirin

Indirect comparisons between drugs are subject to multiple bias, owing to different trial design and population demographics (Table 4.3).

There is so far only one preliminary head-to-head, controlled but not randomized, trial comparing PEG-INF alfa-2b in combination with Ribavirin with PEG-INF alfa-2a in combination with Ribavirin.

In this small sample trial, a higher early and end of treatment response was observed in patients with genotype 1 and 4 receiving PEG-INF alfa-2b versus PEG-INF alfa-2a (Figure 4.17).[54]

A large multicentre trial, Individualized Dosing Efficacy versus flat dosing to Assess optimaL pegylated interferon therapy (IDEAL) is in progress in the US.

Table 4.3 Significant differences in key trials[52,53]

	PEG-IFN alfa-2b	PEG-IFN alfa-2a
Patient populations: US/non-US	68/32%	41/59%
Bridging fibrosis/cirrhosis	29%	12%
Genotype 1 HVL (≤2 million copies/mL)	74%*	61%
Ribavirin dose	800 mg/day	1000–1200 mg/day
Mean weight	82 kg	78.4 kg

*Data on file. Final report: Protocol No. C/198-580.

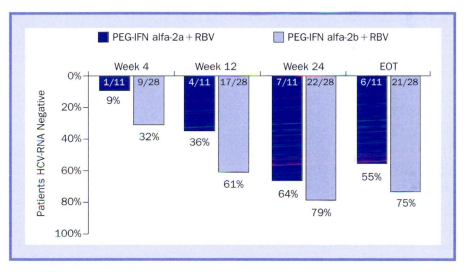

Figure 4.17
Patients HCV-RNA Negative Genotype 1,4

Duration of combination regimen: 12, 24 or 48 weeks?

For a virologic endpoint, the treatment can be stopped at 12 weeks in some subgroups because of a high probability of nonresponse. There were similar results from the three combination trials.[52–55] Among the patients, nongenotype 2 and 3, who had less than a 2-log reduction of baseline viral load at 12 weeks, the probability of a sustained virologic response was less than 5%, despite 48-weeks' treatment. If the HCV-RNA was undetectable at 12 weeks, the percentage of sustained responders was greater than 90%; if the HCV-RNA was still detectable but with a 2-log decrease, 30% of patients became sustained responders.

Before stopping the treatment at 12 weeks,

other factors, such as the antifibrotic effect of treatment in nonresponders or the adherence should be taken into consideration.[56,57]

The choice of 24 or 48 weeks for PEG-IFN and ribavirin combination therapy among the 12-week responders should be clarified. Since patients with many favorable response factors benefit less from 48 weeks of treatment, consideration can be given to stopping at 24 weeks in these patients. A simple strategy could be to consider only the HCV genotype, and stop treatment at week 24 in genotype 2 and 3 responders, since the sustained response was similar in patients treated 24 weeks versus patients treated 48 weeks.[55] However, from our results in the old combination regimens, it seems hazardous to recommend a strategy based only on genotype characteristics. There were, in fact, at least five independent response factors, and to take into account only one factor among these five is an oversimplification that could lead to errors in different populations or subgroups. For example, patients with genotype 2 or 3 who are PCR negative at 24 weeks and who have extensive fibrosis could have better sustained response with 48 weeks of treatment. In patients with genotype 2 and 3 and bridging fibrosis treated with PEG-IFN alfa-2a and ribavirin for 24 weeks, the relapse rate was 18%.[55]

Similarly, patients with genotype 1, with a low level of viremia, younger than 40 and without extensive fibrosis could be treated for only 24 weeks. In the most favorable groups, such as patients with genotype 2 and without bridging fibrosis, perhaps shorter duration therapy could be used.[62]

Steatosis also can be considered as patients with steatosis have lower sustained virological response.[64,65]

Management of relapsers and nonresponders—maintenance therapy

5

Relapsers

A relapser is defined as a patient with HCV RNA that is undetectable in the serum at the end of the treatment but detectable afterwards. When this treatment was interferon, randomized trials have demonstrated that ribavirin interferon in 24 weeks combination permitted clinicians to obtain 55% of sustained response versus 5% in patients retreated by interferon alone.[67]

If relapse occurs after ribavirin interferon combination, the best strategy is to treat with the combination of PEG-IFN and ribavirin adjusted by weight. If relapse occurs after the optimized combination ribavirin interferon, the best strategy is unknown: longer duration or inclusion in randomized trials should be discussed.

Nonresponders

A nonresponder is defined as a patient with still detectable HCV RNA in the serum at the end of the treatment. A nonresponder after interferon alone (24 or 48 weeks) or after the combination ribavirin standard interferon should be treated by the combination of PEG-IFN and ribavirin adjusted by weight.

Maintenance or suppressive therapy

In nonresponders, after the combination of PEG-IFN and ribavirin for at least 24 weeks, the best strategy is unknown.

These patients should be included in randomized trials. If this is not possible, one option is to treat the patients with extensive fibrosis by PEG-IFN alone in order to decrease the progression rate to cirrhosis, while we wait for a new generation of drugs. A small dose of PEG-IFN (that is, 0.5 µg per kg once a week) is interesting in this indication because of its good tolerance and the injection once a week. This concept of maintenance (suppressive therapy) has been developed with standard interferon monotherapy,[8,45,68,69] showing in nonresponders a decrease in fibrosis progression rates (Figure 5.1) and an improvement in necrosis and inflammation (Figure 5.2). Maintenance therapy with interferon should probably be repeated, as after cessation of interferon, fibrosis progression restarted (Figure 5.3). The same effect has been observed with PEG-IFN alone

or in combination with ribavirin among nonresponders.[56,57]

These treatments can reduce the fibrosis progression rate induced by aging. According to Markov age-dependent modeling, a 10-year increment in duration of infection increased the risk of progression by 32% for interferon-treated patients and by 51% for untreated patients. The course of a series of 1000 interferon-treated and 1000 untreated patients was stimulated over 5 years according to the initial stage of fibrosis and age and duration of infection at diagnosis. Interferon treatment decreased the risk of progression to F3 + F4 by a factor of 4.8, for subjects aged 40 years, infected for 10 years, and to F0 + F1 at diagnosis. As age and duration of infection increased, the risk of fibrosis increased and the impact of interferon treatment decreased.[68]

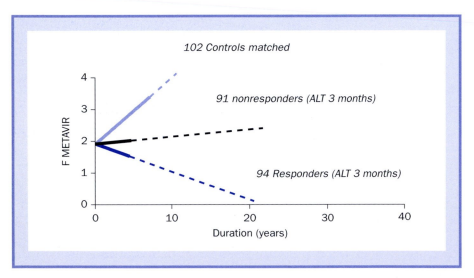

Figure 5.1
Suppressive (or maintenance) concept. Interferon reduces the fibrosis progression among viral nonresponders in comparison with spontaneous progression without treatment. Interferon was given for 24–48 weeks in total, without stopping treatment if ALT was still elevated after 3 months of treatment. Adapted with permission.[8]

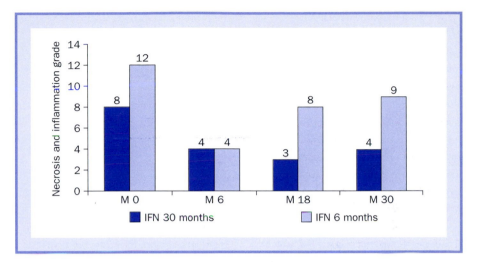

Figure 5.2
Histologic benefit of maintenance therapy with interferon. Virologic nonresponders to six months' interferon were randomized to 24 more months (maintenance therapy n = 27) versus no more treatment (n = 26). There was a significant histologic improvement in patients receiving maintenance therapy. Adapted with permission.[46]

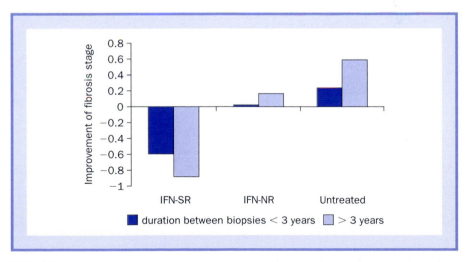

Figure 5.3
Suppressive (or maintenance) concept. Interferon improved the fibrosis stages both in viral responders and in viral nonresponders in comparison with untreated patients. When durations between biopsies were longer than 3 years, the improvement was greater in sustained responders. In viral nonresponders, fibrosis progression restarted after 3 years. In untreated patients, fibrosis progression was time dependent. Adapted with permission.[69]

We pooled individual data from 3010 naive patients with pretreatment and post-treatment biopsies from four randomized trials.[57] Ten different regimens combining standard interferon, PEG-IFN, and ribavirin were compared. The impact of each regimen was estimated by the percentage of patients with at least grade 1 improvement in the necrosis and inflammation (METAVIR score), by the percentage of patients with at least stage 1 worsening in the fibrosis METAVIR score, and by the fibrosis progression rate per year. Necrosis and inflammation improvement ranged from 39% (interferon 24 weeks) to 73% (PEG 1.5 μg/kg plus ribavirin >10.6 mg/kg per day; $p < 0.001$). Fibrosis worsening ranged from 23% (interferon 24 weeks) to 8% (PEG 1.5 μg/kg plus ribavirin >10.6 mg/kg per day; $p < 0.001$). All regimens significantly reduced the fibrosis-progression rates in comparison to rates before treatment. The reversal of cirrhosis was observed in 75 patients (49%) of 153 patients with baseline cirrhosis.

Six factors were independently associated with the absence of significant fibrosis after treatment: baseline fibrosis stage (odds ratio [OR] = 0.12; $p < 0.0001$), sustained viral response (OR = 0.36; $p < 0.0001$), age < 40 years (OR = 0.51; $p < 0.001$), body-mass index < 27 kg/m^2 (OR = 0.65; $p < 0.001$), no or minimal baseline activity (OR = 0.70; $p = 0.02$), and viral load = 3.5 million copies per milliliter (OR = 0.79; $p < 0.03$).

Impact of treatment on hepatocellular carcinoma occurrence and mortality

There is an obvious ethical problem in conducting large randomized trials comparing treatment of chronic hepatitis C (very effective on virologic and histologic endpoints) with placebo in order to prove the reduction of mortality. Retrospective studies controlled or not have shown a decrease in morbidity and mortality in patients treated with interferon.[70–76] The reduction in mortality is significant in patients without sustained virologic response (OR = 0.47; $p = 0.002$) but is higher in patients with a sustained virologic response (OR = 0.15; $p = 0.0001$) and in noncirrhotic patients (OR = 0.36; $p = 0.02$).[76]

Management of patients with cirrhosis

6

Overviews of randomized trials clearly demonstrated that compensated cirrhosis belongs to the full indication of interferon treatment,[45] including PEG-IFN[51,57] and its combinations with ribavirin.[52–57,77]

Although lower than in noncirrhotic patients, there is a significant improvement of interferon monotherapy versus control in randomized trials for ALT response at the end of the treatment (20%), for the sustained ALT response (13%) and for the histologic response, which can reach 80% for 18 months' duration. The effect on HCV RNA seems even better than that observed for ALT. From these results and taking into account the severity of the disease, we think that it is mandatory to treat these patients, as the tolerance is roughly similar to that in noncirrhotic patients. Interferon is able to reduce by 16% the 4-year mortality and by 13% the incidence of hepatocellular carcinoma. The number of randomized studies is small, but the meta-analysis of

Table 6.1 Risk factors for hepatocellular carcinoma in 2400 patients treated by interferon. Adapted with permission.[72]

Type of response to interferon	Risk ratio
Virologic	
Sustained	0.20 p < 0.001
Nonsustained	0.63 p < 0.001
Biochemical ALT	
Sustained	0.20 p < 0.001
Mildly elevated	0.36 p < 0.001
Highly elevated	0.91 NS

controlled retrospective studies with many more patients is impressive, showing the same reduction in hepatocellular carcinoma and mortality[70–76] (Table 6.1).

In patients with cirrhosis, the ribavirin interferon combination achieved a sustained virologic response (below 100 copies per ml 6 months after the end of the treatment) in 20% versus 5% by interferon alone (p = 0.01) (Figure 6.2).[77] The combination of PEG-IFN 1.5 μg per kg and ribavirin in patients with compensated cirrhosis is now logically the new first-line treatment, with a 55% sustained response rate (24 out of 44)[52] (Figure 6.3) and sometimes reversal of cirrhosis.[59] Interferon toxicity on platelets and neutrophils must be carefully monitored.

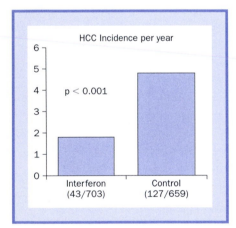

Figure 6.1
Reduction of hepatocellular carcinoma (HCC) incidence following treatment with interferon. Meta-analysis of two randomized controlled trials and five nonrandomized controlled trials of interferon in patients with cirrhosis. Adapted with permission.[51]

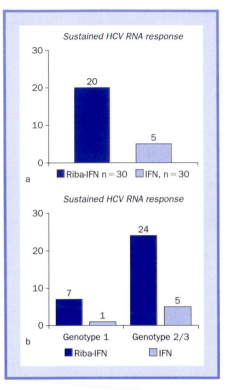

Figure 6.2
Efficacy of ribavirin-interferon (Riba-IFN) therapy in patients with cirrhosis. Patients were given 1–1.2 g ribavirin plus 3 MU interferon alfa-2 TIW, or 3 MU TIW alone. (a) Pivotal randomized trials. (b) Pooled European database. Adapted with permission.[47,48,77]

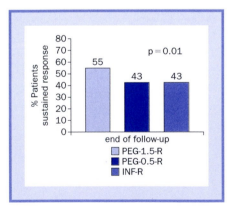

Figure 6.3
Efficacy of optimized combination of PEG-IFN and ribavirin in patients with extensive fibrosis or cirrhosis. Adapted with permission.[52]

Management of patients coinfected by HCV and HIV

7

Among patients infected by HIV, HCV coinfection must be systematically screened (anti-HCV antibodies), and treatment of HCV must be discussed when fibrosis is observed at liver biopsy.[25] When transaminase activity is increased in a patient infected by HIV, a serum HCV PCR must be performed, as false negative of antibodies are possible in immunodepressed patients.

The mean prevalence of HCV antibodies fluctuates between 10% and 30% among large cohorts of patients infected by HIV, is 8% among sexually infected and is 80% among IV drug users.

An increase in survival of HIV-infected persons related to active antiretroviral therapies highlights the problem of chronic hepatitis C. The prevalence of cirrhosis is threefold higher in HIV-HCV-coinfected patients than in HIV-negative HCV-infected patients, and one-third of coinfected patients are at risk of dying of liver disease.[25]

The progression of fibrosis is more rapid in coinfected patients than in matched controls infected by HCV alone. In coinfected patients, a low CD4 count ($\leq$200 cells/μL), alcohol consumption ($>$50 g/day) and age at HCV infection are associated with a higher liver fibrosis progression rate.[19,24,25,26]

Anti-HIV treatment is often associated with an increase in transaminases (D4T, DDI, abacavir, nevirapine and protease inhibitor). When the increase is important, another liver biopsy (or biochemical markers) must be discussed and compared to biopsy (or biochemical markers) before treatment. The following factors can be involved: alcohol consumption, illicit IV drug injection, substitution drug toxicity, anti-HIV drug toxicity, coinfection with HBV or delta virus, liver opportunistic infection, immune restoration and sclerosing cholangitis. The impact of immune reconstitution on liver fibrosis progression is unknown. However, we have observed a slower fibrosis progression rate in patients receiving antiprotease than in patients not receiving antiprotease. This difference persisted after adjustment by confounding factors.[78]

According to the very severe natural history, the most effective treatment of hepatitis C should be given to coinfected patients. Results and tolerance are lower than those of patients infected by HCV only, but the benefit-risk ratio is probably identical or even higher.[25,79]

Discussion of hepatitis C treatment in a patient coinfected by HIV and HCV

1. If the patient is not treated for HIV and there is no indication for this treatment, a treatment by the ribavirin and PEG-IFN combination should be discussed, as there is a high risk of fibrosis progression.

2. If the patient is not treated for HIV and there is an indication for this treatment, the treatment of HIV must be given without concomitant treatment of HCV. Treatment of HCV can start 6 months later after a good immune and HIV response.

3. If the patient is under treatment for HIV, the treatment of HCV can start when a good immune and HIV response has been obtained.

4. If a patient has a very rapid progression of liver fibrosis with a risk of cirrhosis at short term, the treatment of HCV should be discussed in association with anti-HIV treatment, even if the response to HIV treatment is partial.

5. Alcohol consumption should be prohibited in all coinfected HIV-HCV patients because of the rapid fibrosis progression to cirrhosis.

Management of HCV infection after liver transplantation

8

Cirrhosis due to HCV is with alcoholic cirrhosis the most common indication for orthotopic liver transplantation (OLT) worldwide. After OLT, HCV RNA universally reappears with detectable HCV RNA, and 50–80% of transplant recipients develop clinical graft hepatitis,[80] with probably a more rapid fibrosis progression rate than in nontransplanted patients.[81] Donor age has a major influence on graft outcome following transplantation.[81,82]

There is a consensus for treating patients with recurrence and fibrosis progression and to reduce immunosuppressive therapy. After recurrence, the combination of interferon and ribavirin is effective with an acceptable tolerance,[83–86] and combination with PEG-IFN should increase this efficacy. There is probably an increased risk of hemolysis and anemia associated with ribavirin in these patients.[85]

There are no clearly defined markers with high predictive values to identify candidates for prophylactic treatment. Interferon monotherapy is effective for prevention of recurrence[86] (Figure 8.1), and PEG-IFN and ribavirine trials are needed, according to an encouraging pilot trial of the combination[87] (Table 8.1). Liver transplantation is effective in selected HIV-positive patients suffering from end-stage liver disease.[88] Patient and graft survival are similar to non-HIV-positive patients suffering from the same indications. Given the complex pharmacologic interactions between the protease inhibitors and tacrolimus, careful monitoring and attention are required to prevent toxicity or underdosing.[88]

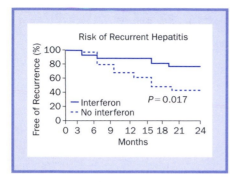

Figure 8.1
Efficacy of interferon alfa-2b in the prophylaxis of recurrent hepatitis C after liver transplantation. Adapted with permission.[86]

Table 8.1 A pilot trial of the combination ribavirin and interferon alfa-2b in the prophylaxis of recurrent hepatitis C after liver transplantation. Adapted with permission.[87] Twenty-one patients were included (19 genotype 1b) and were treated within 3 weeks of transplantation and for 48 weeks.

Clinical events	No. of patients
Acute graft hepatitis	4
Persistent hepatitis	3
Chronic active hepatitis	1
Cirrhosis	0
No evidence of hepatitis	17 (81%)
HCV RNA seroconversion	9 (41%)
1-year survival	95%
Dose reduction	43%

Management of patients with renal disease

9

Hepatitis C virus is frequent in patients with end-stage renal disease. HCV infection continues to occur in dialysis patients because of nosocomial spread. HCV infection affects the survival of chronic dialysis patients as well as renal transplant recipients.[89] The severity of liver disease on pretransplantation liver biopsy, or on biochemical markers, provides useful prognostic information after renal transplantation. There are only limited data about interferon or PEG-IFN therapy in chronic dialysis patients, although sustained responses are reported. Preliminary data on the interferon and ribavirin combination in dialysis patients with hepatitis C have given encouraging results.[90] Six patients were given interferon alfa-2b 3 MU thrice weekly for 4 weeks, after which ribavirin 200–400 mg was added, for an intended total treatment period of 28 weeks. Ribavirin plasma concentrations were monitored by HPLC. Four patients completed the treatment. According to plasma concentrations, ribavirin doses were frequently adjusted initially. The target concentration (10–15 μmol/L) was reached with average daily doses of 170–300 mg ribavirin. Ribavirin-induced anemia was managed with high doses of erythropoietin (20 000–30 000 IU/week). Five of six patients became hepatitis C virus (HCV)-RNA negative during treatment, but four relapsed after treatment; one was HCV-RNA negative. This regimen requires reduced ribavirin doses and close monitoring of ribavirin plasma concentrations and hemoglobin. Interferon remains contraindicated in post-renal transplantation because of concern about precipitating graft dysfunction. Ribavirin alone can be used, but the benefit-risk ratio is unknown.

Other difficult-to-treat populations

10

Management of hemophiliac patients

Most hemophiliac patients were infected with hepatitis C virus through transfusion with contaminated plasma and plasma products before the mid-1980s, and about 80% became chronically infected.[91] The natural history, after taking into account the age at infection and the possible HIV coinfection, is similar to that in nonhemophiliac subjects. In the absence of treatment, approximately 20% of people with chronic HCV infection will progress to severe liver disease, such as cirrhosis, end-stage liver diseases or hepatocellular carcinoma.[92] As in nonhemophiliacs, the fibrosis progression rate is increased in patients coinfected with HIV.[92,93]

The management of hepatitis C in hemophiliac patients is similar to that in nonhemophiliac patients,[93–95] including liver transplantation.[94] An important difference is the cost-benefit ratio of liver biopsy. Because of coagulation defects, there are no consensual recommendations for the liver biopsy indication and procedures.[96–100] Studies included very small numbers of patients, and the risk is not known. The cost of biopsy is much higher than in the nonhemophiliac population if hemophiliac patients must be hospitalized with factor infusion.[100]

Management of thalassemic patients

More than 80% of transfusion-dependent thalassemic patients are infected by HCV.[101] The natural history of fibrosis progression is probably more rapid than in nonthalassemic patients because of the iron overload and the insulin resistance.[101] However, the management was similar to that of nonthalassemic patients when interferon was the standard regimen. With ribavirin and interferon combination, transfusions are sometimes needed during treatment, but the overall sustained-response rates are similar to those in nonthalassemic patients.[102–106] Bone marrow transplantation is not a contraindication to subsequent treatment of chronic hepatitis C.[106]

Management of patients with anemia, neutropenia and thrombocytopenia

Anemia, neutropenia and thrombocytopenia are major hematologic toxicities of therapy. These effects are generally managed with dose reductions and are reversible upon treatment discontinuation. Emerging evidence suggests that early initiation of growth factors may allow patients to remain on higher doses, allowing greater antiviral efficacy.

Ribavirin induces a dose-dependent, reversible hemolytic anemia (Figure 11.1). Erythropoietin (epoetin alfa) therapy may be an effective treatment for ribavirin-induced anemia.[107,108] The cost-effectiveness of epoetin has been demonstrated in cancer patients but is not yet clearly established for chronic hepatitis C. The rationale for treatment is that the fatigue produced by interferon and ribavirin-related anemia is associated with reduced quality of life. Moreover, anemia may result in severe adverse events, in a need of blood transfusion and in failure to meet treatment-adherence goals. The mean hemoglobin drop observed in a small randomized trial was 2.9 g/dL in the standard of care group and 0.3 g/dL in the group receiving 40 000 units/week.[108] At week 16, the mean daily doses of ribavirin were 700 and 900, respectively. Therefore, if epoetin is started before the hemoglobin level drops below 11 g/dL, a ribavirin dose reduction can be avoided. Patients who are anemic at baseline can be started on epoetin prior to treatment. Normal iron stores are needed for an adequate response to epoetin.

Patients with baseline neutropenia or who develop neutropenia during therapy can be treated with granulocyte colony-stimulating factor (G-CSF). G-CSF potentiates the effect of epoetin.[109,110] The usual dose is 300 µg administered subcutaneously once to thrice weekly and then titrated to maintain an absolute neutrophil count above 750. Adverse events include skin rash, vasculitis, bone pain, myalgia, thrombocytopenia, splenomegaly, leukemoid reaction and exacerbation of psoriasis.

Thrombocytopenia is mainly problematic in cirrhotic patients with portal hypertension and spleen enlargement. In noncirrhotic patients, a severe decrease is exceptional. Interleukin-11, which is used in cancer patients, has been studied in HCV-infected patients.[111] Platelets increased 5–9 days after subcutaneous injection (25–50 µg IL-11). Potential adverse events include edema, fluid retention, dyspnea, atrial arrhythmia and dilutional anemia. There is no interaction with G-CSF or epoietin.

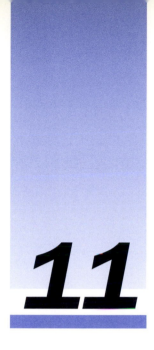

Safety of interferon, pegylated interferon (PEG-IFN) and ribavirin

11

Patients should be fully informed of the potential adverse events before starting therapy.[112]

Safety of standard interferon and ribavirin

Severe adverse events

For interferon, the main severe adverse events are depression, suicidal ideation, suicide and sustained hypothyroidism. For ribavirin, the main severe adverse events are anemia and teratogenic effects. There is a 3 g/dL mean drop in hemoglobin concentration in the first 4 weeks of treatment (Figure 11.1). Blood cell count must be checked at least 2 and 4 weeks after starting therapy and every 4 weeks thereafter. In case of hemoglobin lower than 10 g/dL, ribavirin should be reduced by 50%. If hemoglobin is lower than 8 g/dL, ribavirin should be stopped.

Frequent adverse events (Table 11.1)

For interferon, the most frequent adverse events are flu-like symptoms and alopecia. For ribavirin, the most frequent adverse event is anemia; less frequently, we have pharyngitis, insomnia, dyspnea, pruritus, rash, nausea and anorexia.

Uncommon and rare adverse events

Side effects occurring in less than 2% of patients treated by combination therapy include autoimmune disease (especially

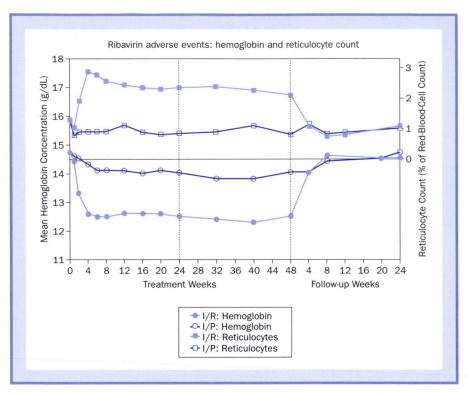

Figure 11.1
Impact of ribavirin-interferon on hemoglobin and reticulocyte count in patients treated by interferon and ribavirin.

thyroid disease), severe bacterial infections, marked neutropenia, seizures, retinopathy with microhemorrhages, hearing loss and tinnitus.

Contraindications to treatment

Contraindications to interferon alfa therapy include psychosis, severe depression, active substance or alcohol abuse, severe heart disease, severe neutropenia or thrombocytopenia, organ transplantation (except liver), decompensated cirrhosis, uncontrolled seizures, pregnancy, and nonreliable method of contraception. In fact,

with the advice of a psychiatrist, it is sometimes possible to treat patients with psychosis or depression. Patients with bone-marrow compromise or cytopenia (neutrophils <1000 and <75 000 platelet count per mm³) should be treated cautiously with frequent monitoring of cell counts. Relative contraindications are uncontrolled diabetes and uncontrolled autoimmune disorders, such as rheumatoid arthritis, lupus erythematosus, psoriasis and thyroiditis.

Absolute contraindications to ribavirin are pregnancy, nonreliable method of contraception, end-stage renal failure, severe

Table 11.1 Adverse events (%) observed in the nonpegylated interferon and ribavirin combination randomized trials.

	24 weeks		48 weeks	
	Interferon/ ribavirin	Interferon /placebo	Interferon/ ribavirin	Interferon/ placebo
Discontinuation for adverse events	8	9	21	14
Dose reduction for anemia	7	0	9	0
Dose reduction for other adverse events	13	12	17	9
Flu-like symptoms				
Fatigue	68	62	70	72
Headache	63	63	67	66
Myalgia	61	57	64	63
Fever	37	35	41	40
Arthralgia	30	27	33	36
Musculoskeletal pain	20	26	28	32
Psychiatric symptoms				
Insomnia	39	27	39	30
Depression	32	25	36	37
Irritability	23	19	32	27
Impaired concentration	11	14	14	14
Anxiety	10	9	18	13
Suicidal ideation	0.6	0.4	2.6	0.2
Attempted suicide	0.2	0	0.2	0
Gastrointestinal symptoms				
Nausea	38	35	46	33
Anorexia	27	16	25	19
Diarrhea	18	22	22	26
Abdominal pain	15	17	14	20
Dyspepsia	14	6	16	9
Dermatologic symptoms				
Alopecia	28	27	32	28
Pruritus	21	9	19	8
Rash	20	9	28	8
Inflammation at injection site	13	10	12	14
Respiratory tract symptoms				
Dyspnea	19	9	18	10
Cough	15	5	14	9
Pharyngitis	11	9	20	10

anemia and hemoglobinopathies. Relative contraindications are medical conditions in which anemia can be dangerous, especially coronary heart disease and cerebrovascular disease. Fatal myocardial infarctions and strokes have been reported during combination therapy. Patients with pre-existing hemolysis or anemia (hemoglobin <11 g per dL) should not receive ribavirin.

Safety of PEG-IFN and ribavirin

The adverse event profiles of PEG-IFN alfa-2b or alfa-2a plus ribavirin and standard interferon plus ribavirin were similar. There were no new or unique adverse events, and the tolerance of different kinds of PEG-IFN was similar, with the same percentage of severe adverse events[52–55,112] (Table 11.2).

There was an increased incidence (greater than 5%) of flu-like symptoms with PEG-IFN compared to standard interferon, as well as

Table 11.2 Common adverse events (at least 10%) observed in the PEG-IFN alfa-2b and ribavirin combination randomized trial. Adapted with permission.[52]

	48 weeks	
	PEG-interferon 1.5/ ribavirin n = 511	Interferon 3 MU TIW/ ribavirin n = 505
Discontinuation for adverse events	14	13
Dose reduction for anemia	9	13
Dose reduction for neutropenia	18	8
Dose reduction for all reasons	42	34
Flu-like symptoms		
Fatigue	64	60
Headache	62	58
Myalgia	56	48
Fever	46	33
Arthralgia	34	28
Musculoskeletal pain	21	19
Psychiatric symptoms		
Insomnia	40	41
Depression	31	34
Irritability	35	34
Impaired concentration	17	21
Anxiety	15	15
Gastrointestinal symptoms		
Nausea	43	33
Anorexia	32	27
Diarrhea	22	17
Abdominal pain	13	13
Vomiting	14	12
Dermatologic symptoms		
Alopecia	36	32
Pruritus	29	28
Rash	24	23
Inflammation at injection site	25	18
Respiratory tract symptoms		
Dyspnea	26	24
Cough	17	13
Pharyngitis	12	13

neutropenia. As previously reported with PEG-IFN monotherapy, there was a significant increase in injection-site reaction. This reaction was generally mild, with localized erythema, and was not treatment limiting.

The impact of ribavirin dose optimization according to the weight was minor,[52] with few more frequent adverse events (>5% difference) in the optimized group of asthenia, cough and alopecia.

A decrease in hemoglobin to less than 10 g/dL occurred in 14% of patients receiving the optimized combination. A dose reduction for neutropenia (less than 750×10^9/L) occurred in 21% of patients receiving the optimized combination, with less than 1% of discontinuation (less than 500×10^9/L). The impact on hemoglobin, neutrophil and platelet counts was maximum in the first 4 weeks (Figures 11.1 and 11.2).

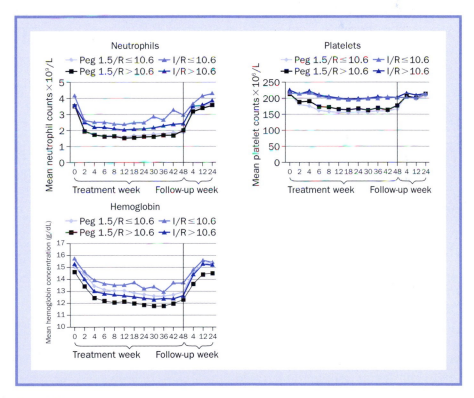

Figure 11.2
Impact of the optimized PEG-IFN and ribavirin combination on neutrophils, platelets and hemoglobin. Adapted with permission.[52]

Who needs to be treated and how to explain the goals to the patient

12

An algorithm for treatment decision is presented in Figure 12.1. Considering the natural history of hepatitis C, there are three different goals of the treatment: (1) to prevent the occurrence of cirrhosis and its complications, (2) to reduce the extrahepatic manifestations and (3) to prevent the infection of other people (that is, surgeon or drug user).

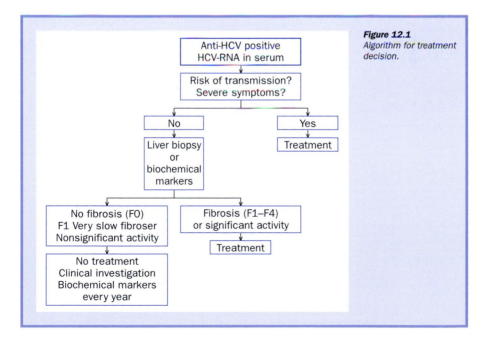

Figure 12.1
Algorithm for treatment decision.

Is there a group of patients for whom the treatment is useless?

If the patient is not at risk of progress to cirrhosis, has no symptom, and is not at risk of transmitting the virus, there is no need to treat (for example, a 60-year-old asymptomatic subject contaminated 30 years ago and without fibrosis at biopsy). Patients without fibrosis (METAVIR F0) represent only 7% of a study on 4552 patients.

If the patient has decompensated cirrhosis, the benefit of treatment is unknown. Because of adverse events, particularly leukopenia, interferon and ribavirin are not presently recommended. Prospective trials are needed in these patients, especially before transplantation.

How to explain the treatment

An "a la carte" regimen can be explained and discussed with patients according to their own response factors (Figure 16.1). The major risk of adverse events during follow-up and the consequences for interferon and ribavirin doses must be explained (Figure 16.2).

What is the cost-effectiveness of combination regimens?

13

The treatment of hepatitis C is effective and costly. Hepatitis C and its complications are even more costly. Therefore, combination regimens are cost-effective as compared with other widely accepted medical interventions.[113–116] Compared with no antiviral therapy, PEG-IFN plus weight-based dosing of ribavirin increased life expectancy by 4.7 years. Compared with standard interferon alfa-2b plus ribavirin, PEG-IFN plus weight-based dosing of ribavirin increased life expectancy by 1.0 year with incremental cost-effectiveness ratios of 6600 euros per quality-adjusted life year (QALY), respectively. Subgroup analyses by genotype, viral load, sex, and histology showed that PEG-IFN plus weight-based ribavirin remained cost-effective compared with other well-accepted medical treatments (Tables 13.1–13.5).

Table 13.1 Direct medical cost of diagnosis.

Diagnostic test	Cost in euros From mean French prices	Cost in US dollars From US government mean reimbursement prices (private prices)
ALT	7	9
ELISA	20	27
HCV PCR	40	37
Viral load	70	80 (150)
Genotype	100	200 (250)
Liver ultrasonography	60	100 (240)
FibroTest-ActiTest	90	85 (not approved)
Liver biopsy	700	370 (1000)

Table 13.2 Base case analysis: life expectancy, quality-adjusted life expectancy, and direct lifetime costs discounted at 3%. Adapted with permission.[95]

	No antiviral treatment	Interferon plus ribavirin	PEG-IFN plus fixed ribavirin	PEG-IFN plus weight-based ribavirin
Cost €	14 100	19 300	21 800	22 400
Life expectancy (years)	17.0	18.6	18.8	19.1
Quality-adjusted life expectancy (years)	15.1	16.8	17.0	17.3

Table 13.3 Direct medical cost of disease (office visits, laboratory tests, medications other than interferon or ribavirin, hospitalizations). Adapted with permission.[116]

Disease	Annual costs in euros
Chronic hepatitis without cirrhosis	130
Noncomplicated cirrhosis	673
Complicated cirrhosis sensitive ascites	1914
Hepatic encephalopathy (first year)	7738
Variceal hemorrhage (first year)	12 314
Diuretic refractory ascites	12 534
Hepatocellular carcinoma	17 244
Transplantation (first year)	117 303

Table 13.4 Cost-effectiveness of combination therapy: comparison of cost and gain in life expectancy versus coronary artery bypass surgery. Adapted with permission.[115]

	Cost €	Gain in life expectancy
PEG-IFN plus weight-based ribavirin	22 400	2.1 years
Coronary artery bypass surgery	27 000	1.1 years

Table 13.5 Cost-effectiveness of combination therapy: comparison of cost per quality-adjusted life years versus accepted medical interventions. Adapted with permission.[115]

	Incremental cost per quality-adjusted life years (€)
PEG-IFN plus weight-based ribavirin	6600
Screening blood donors for HIV	14 000
Treatment of hypertension (70-year-old)	5300
Coronary artery bypass	60 000
Treatment of hypertension (40-year-old)	85 000

Management of acute hepatitis C

14

Spontaneous clearance of acute hepatitis C

Because of the small number of patients analyzed, the factors associated with spontaneous clearance of serum HCV RNA and acute hepatitis C cure have not been well identified. The percentage of patients with spontaneous viral clearance varies from 4% to 30%.[117-121] Patients with jaundice have more spontaneous clearance than asymptomatic patients. One explanation is that there is a better immune response in patients with jaundice than patients without symptoms. There is no clear predictive value for the viral load or the genotype. As expected, patients without a rapid decrease in viral load are at higher risk of chronicity than patients without viral load decrease. Almost all spontaneous clearances occur 24 weeks after the infection; that is, 12 weeks after the occurrence of symptoms. Viral quasispecies' diversity has also been associated with the occurrence of chronicity in comparison with a homogeneous viral population.

Treatment of acute hepatitis C

Overviews of randomized or nonrandomized trials have shown that interferon alone has a high effectiveness in comparison to control groups.[120,121]

Six randomized trials involving 206 patients with acute hepatitis were included in a meta-analysis, four trials assessing interferon alfa-2b in 141 patients, all with transfusion-acquired acute hepatitis C. When compared with no treatment, interferon alfa-2b was associated with an increase in the rates of virologic end-of-treatment response and sustained response by 45% (95% CI 31–59%, p < 0.00001) and 29% (95% CI 14–44%, p = 0.0002), respectively. At the end of follow-up, a virologic response was seen in 32% (95% CI 21–46%) of interferon-treated patients versus only 4% (95% CI 0–13%, p = 0.00007) of controls.

Because of the small number of symptomatic patients, randomized trials are not a rapid method to identify a new regimen in acute hepatitis C. A multicenter study included 44 patients, who received 5 million units of interferon alfa-2b subcutaneously daily for 4 weeks and then three times per week for another 20 weeks.[121] Serum HCV-RNA levels were measured before and during therapy and 24 weeks after the end of therapy. The average time from infection to the first signs or symptoms of hepatitis was 54 days,

and the average time from infection until the start of therapy was 89 days. At the end of both therapy and follow-up, 43 patients (98%) had undetectable levels of HCV RNA in serum and normal serum alanine aminotransferase levels. Levels of HCV RNA became undetectable after an average of 3.2 weeks of treatment. Therapy was well tolerated in all but one patient, who stopped therapy after 12 weeks because of side effects.

Therefore, a regimen with a high dose of interferon alfa for 24 weeks can be recommended in the treatment of acute hepatitis C. The benefit-risk ratio of PEG-IFN alone or in combination with ribavirin is unknown.

The treatment could be started 12 weeks after jaundice if the HCV RNA is still detectable. In patients without jaundice, a treatment can be discussed earlier according to the high risk of chronicity and the high effectiveness of interferon.

Practical guidelines for the management of hepatitis C

15

Liver biopsy and biochemical markers of fibrosis and necrosis

Polymerase chain reaction (PCR) HCV RNA testing establishes the diagnosis of hepatitis C infection. Assessing the histologic features, by liver biopsy or biochemical markers,[122,123] is helpful before treating a patient, for the decision and the duration of therapy. The estimation of histologic features includes staging the severity of disease (fibrosis stage) and grading the amount of necrosis and inflammation.

Biopsy is also helpful in ruling out other causes of liver disease such as alcoholic features, nonalcoholic steatohepatitis, autoimmune hepatitis, medication-induced, coinfection with HBV or HIV, or iron overload. Liver biopsy is usually performed by the intercostal route. In clotting disorders, the transjugular route is used. The limits and advantages of biopsy and biochemical markers are discussed in Section III.

PCR amplification

With the latest methods, PCR can detect 10–50 IU/ml of HCV RNA. Testing for HCV RNA is a reliable way of demonstrating HCV infection and is the most specific test of infection. Testing HCV RNA is particularly useful when transaminases are normal, when several causes of liver disease are possible (such as alcohol consumption), in immunosuppressed patients (that is, after transplantation, in

HIV-coinfected patients) and in acute hepatitis C before occurrence of antibodies (4–10 weeks).

Enzyme immunoassay

Anti-HCV is detected by enzyme immunoassay. The third-generation test is usually very sensitive and very specific. In the case of false-positive or false-negative doubts, the best test for confirmation of HCV infection is HCV RNA PCR. Immunosuppressed patients infected by HCV may test negative for anti-HCV. Antibody is usually present by 1 month (4–10 weeks) after onset of acute illness. Anti-HCV is still detectable during and after treatment, whatever the response, and must not be tested again.

Genotype and serotype

There are six genotypes of hepatitis C and more than 50 subtypes. Knowing genotype or serotype (genotype-specific antibodies) is helpful for the pegylated or not interferon-ribavirin treatment duration choice. Genotypes do not change during the course of infection and must not be tested again. Knowing subtypes (that is, 1a versus 1b) is not clinically helpful. There is no relationship between the severity of the disease (fibrosis stage) and genotypes.

Quantification of HCV RNA in serum

Methods measuring the level of virus in serum use quantitative PCR and the branched DNA (bDNA) test. They are currently less sensitive than qualitative assays.

An effort has been made to define clinically relevant HCV-RNA loads in standardized international units (IU), for use in routine clinical and research applications based on standardized quantitative assays validated with appropriately calibrated panels.[124] The semiautomated quantitative RT-PCR Superquant assay (National Genetics Institute, Los Angeles, CA) has a range from 50 to 1 470 000 IU/mL; the semiautomated Cobas Amplicor HCV Monitor assay version 2.0 (Cobas v2.0, Roche Molecular Systems, Pleasanton, CA) has a range from 600 to 2 630 000 IU/mL; the semiautomated HCV RNA quantitative assay LCx (Abbott Diagnostics, Chicago, IL) has a range of 25 to 2 630 000 IU/ml; the semiautomated branched DNA signal amplification Versant HCV RNA 3.0 assay (bDNA) (Bayer Corporation, Diagnostic Division, Tarrytown, NY) has a range of 615 to 7 700 000 IU/mL; the manual branched DNA signal amplification (Quantiplex) Versant HCV RNA 2.0 assay (bDNA) (Bayer Corporation, Diagnostic Division, Tarrytown, NY) has a range of 3200 to 19 000 000 IU/mL.

In the more recent studies, the median of viral load ranged from 800 000 IU/mL (5.9 $\log_{10}$ IU/mL) to nearly 1 300 000 IU/mL (6.1 $\log_{10}$ IU/mL).

Knowing the viral load is helpful for the pegylated or not interferon-ribavirin treatment duration choice. Patients with high initial viral load have higher relapse rates and benefit more from a 48-week regimen than patients with lower viral load. A 12-week stopping rule is also possible when the viral load decrease is less than 2 logs in comparison with baseline value. Unlike HIV infection, viral load does not correlate to severity of hepatitis (fibrosis progression).

HCV-core antigen assays

HCV-core antigen can be detected in the serum and quantified (Total HCV-core antigen assay, Ortho-Clinical Diagnostics, Raritan, USA). This quantification can be used as an indirect marker of the HCV viral load, but it is less sensitive than molecular HCV-RNA assays.[125]

Ten key points for patients' understanding of the natural history

1. Almost all the mortality of the disease is related to complications of cirrhosis.
2. There is hardly ever a spontaneous clearance of the virus in chronic hepatitis.
3. One-third of infected patients will probably never progress to cirrhosis. One-third will progress without treatment in around 30 years, and one-third will progress in less than 20 years.
4. Despite the risk of fibrosis, a patient can be treated for extrahepatic manifestations or in order to prevent transmission of the virus.
5. Cryoglobulinemia is very common (40%) and is rarely associated with severe symptoms (1% of vasculitis).
6. The viral load and genotype are not related to the severity of the disease.
7. Alcohol consumption greater than four units a day accelerates the fibrosis progression.
8. Aging accelerates the fibrosis progression, particularly after 50 years of age.

9. HIV coinfection and immunosuppression accelerate the fibrosis progression.
10. Normal transaminases do not exclude a progression to cirrhosis even if the risk is less than among patients with elevated transamines.

Ten key points for patients' understanding of the treatment

1. There are two goals for the treatment of hepatic manifestation: the first goal is to eradicate the virus; if the virus is not eradicated, the second goal is to prevent the progression to cirrhosis and the complications of cirrhosis.
2. When a sustained viral response is obtained (negative PCR 3 months after the end of treatment), the late relapse rate is lower than 5% 4 years later.
3. When a sustained viral response is obtained, there is a dramatic improvement of liver histology, including necroinflammatory features and fibrosis stage.
4. When a sustained viral response is obtained in cirrhotic patients, a few randomized trials and several retrospective studies have observed that the incidence of complications is decreased in comparison to nontreated patients.
5. When a sustained viral response is not obtained, there is a controversy concerning the benefit of treatment. Randomized trials and modeling have shown in these patients an improvement of transaminase activity, viral load,

necroinflammatory lesions and fibrosis progression in comparison to the natural history.

6. The long-term impact of treatment on extrahepatic manifestations is unknown. The health-related quality of life is improved after treatment in sustained responders.

7. During treatment, the quality of life of the patient is generally worse than before due to the adverse events, but it improves thereafter in sustained responders.

8. Depression and suicide are the most dreadful adverse events of interferon.

9. Anemia and teratogenicity are the most dreadful adverse events of ribavirin.

10. After treatment, all adverse events disappeared, with the exception of dysthyroidia, in less than 3%.

New drugs in development

16

The most interesting drugs in development are the small molecules, inhibitors of the HCV enzymes of virus replication: protease, helicase and polymerase. An oral HCV serine protease inhibitor (BILN 2061, Boehringer Ingelheim Pharma KG, Biberach, Germany) was administered to 31 patients of genotype 1 without extensive fibrosis (25, 200 and 500 mg) over 2 days versus placebo in an open sequential group comparison.[126] Viral load decreased by at least 1 log in 25 out of 26 treated patients, and no response was observed in five patients receiving the placebo. Viral load returned to baseline levels within 1–7 days. In another randomized, double-blind comparison, 10 patients of genotype 1 with extensive fibrosis, but without decompensated cirrhosis, were treated orally with 200 mg BILN 2061 or placebo over 2 days. Viral load decreased by at least 2 logs in 8/8 patients treated and 0/2 in the placebo group (Figure 16.3). Analysis of adverse events, vital signs, routine laboratory tests and ECG did not reveal relevant drug-induced changes in any of these 34 treated patients.

Other drugs include new immune modulators, new ribavirin analogs deprived of hematologic toxicity, ribozymes and antisense molecules.

The development of an effective HCV vaccine has so far been disappointing.[129] The immunologic correlates of recovery from HCV infection are partially understood. HCV is highly heterogeneous and escapes from the host immune response by rapid mutation. There are no suitable small animal models and cell-culture systems to study HCV

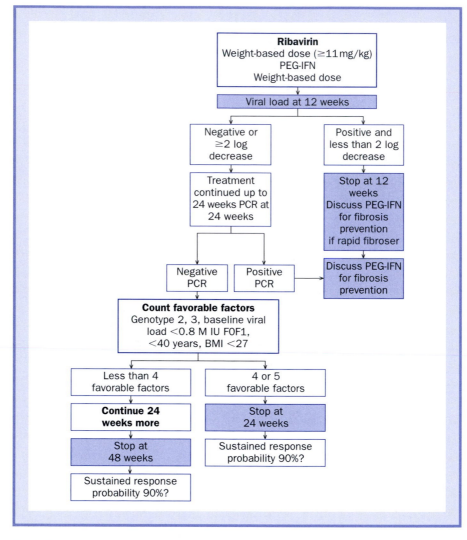

Figure 16.1
Proposed treatment regimen algorithm according to response factors.

infection and replication. The neutralizing
antibodies produced in acute infection do not
provide protection against subsequent
exposure.

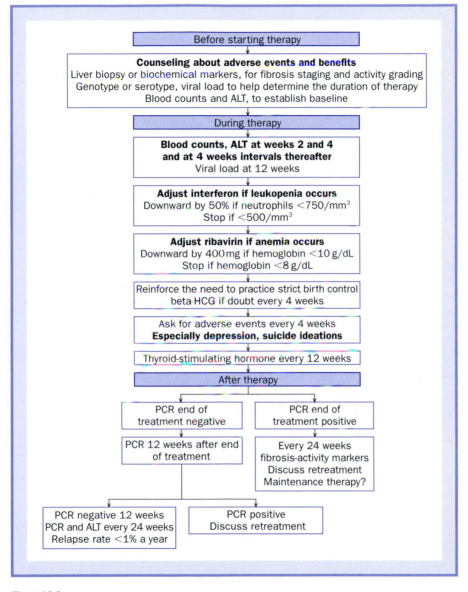

Figure 16.2
Proposed follow-up of treated patients.

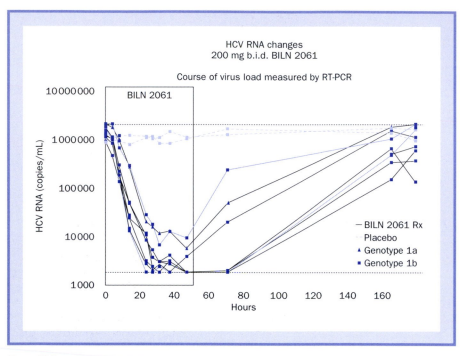

Figure 16.3
Efficacy of BILN 2061 in chronic hepatitis C genotype 1.
Adapted with permission.[127]

References

1. WHO. Hepatitis C: Global prevalence. *Wkly Epidemiol Rec* 1997; **72**: 341–4.

2. Darby SC, Ewart DW, Giangrande PLF, et al. Mortality from liver cancer and liver disease in haemophilic men and boys given blood products contaminated with hepatitis C. *Lancet* 1997; **350**: 1425–31.

3. El-Serag HB, Mason A. Rising incidence of hepatocellular carcinoma in the United States. *N Engl J Med* 1999; **34**: 745–50.

4. Deuffic S, Buffat L, Poynard T, Valleron AJ. Modeling the hepatitis C virus epidemic in France. *Hepatology* 1999; **29**: 1596–601.

5. Deuffic S, Poynard T, Valleron AJ. Correlation between HCV prevalence and hepatocellular carcinoma mortality in Europe. *J Viral Hepat* 1999; **6**: 411–13.

6. Alter MJ, Kruszon-Moran D, Nainan OV, et al. The prevalence of hepatitis C virus infection in the United States, 1988 through 1994. *N Engl J Med* 1999; **341**: 556–62.

7. Poynard T, Bedossa P, Opolon P, for the OBSVIRC, METAVIR, CLINIVIR and DOSVIRC groups. Natural history of liver fibrosis progression in patients with chronic hepatitis C. *Lancet* 1997; **349**: 825–32.

8. Sobesky R, Mathurin P, Charlotte F, et al. Modeling the impact of interferon alfa treatment on liver fibrosis progression in chronic hepatitis C: A dynamic view. *Gastroenterology* 1999; **116**: 378–86.

9. Knodell KG, Ishak KG, Black WC, et al. Formulation and application of a numerical scoring system for assessing histological activity in asymptomatic chronic active hepatitis. *Hepatology* 1981; **1**: 431–5.

10. Ishak K, Baptista A, Bianchi L, et al. Histological grading and

staging of chronic hepatitis. *J Hepatol* 1995; 22: 696–9.

11. METAVIR Cooperative Group. Inter- and intra-observer variation in the assessment of liver biopsy of chronic hepatitis C. *Hepatology* 1994; **20**: 15–20.

12. Bedossa P, Poynard T. An algorithm for the grading of activity in chronic hepatitis C. METAVIR Cooperative Study Group. *Hepatology* 1996; **24**: 289–93.

13. Paradis V, Mathurin P, Laurent A, et al. Histological features predictive of liver fibrosis in chronic hepatitis C infection. *J Clin Pathol* 1996; **49**: 998–1004.

14. Yano M, Kumada H, Kage M, et al. The long-term pathological evolution of chronic hepatitis C. *Hepatology* 1996; **23**: 1334–40.

15. Datz C, Cramp M, Haas T, et al. The natural course of hepatitis C virus infection 18 years after an epidemic outbreak of non-A, non-B hepatitis in a plasmapheresis centre. *Gut* 1999; **44**: 563–7.

16. Poynard T, Ratziu V, Charlotte F, et al. Rates and risk factors of liver fibrosis progression in patients with chronic hepatitis C. *J Hepatol* 2001; **34**: 730–9.

17. Ghany MG, Kleiner DE, Alter H, et al. Progression of fibrosis in chronic hepatitis C. *Gastroenterology* 2003; **124**: 97–104.

18. Wiley TE, McCarthy M, Breidi L, McCarthy M, Layden TJ. Impact of alcohol on the histological and clinical progression of hepatitis C infection. *Hepatology* 1998; **28**: 805–9.

19. Benhamou Y, Bochet M, Di Martino V, et al. Liver fibrosis progression in human immunodeficiency virus and hepatitis C virus coinfected patients. The Multivirc Group. *Hepatology* 1999; **30**: 1054–8.

20. Bissell DM. Sex and hepatic fibrosis. *Hepatology* 1999; **29**: 988–9.

21. Hourigan LF, Macdonald GA, Purdie D, et al. Fibrosis in chronic hepatitis C correlates significantly with body mass index and steatosis. *Hepatology* 1999; **29**: 1215–19.

22. Ortiz V, Berenguer M, Rayon JM, Carrasco D, Berenguer J. Contribution of obesity to hepatitis C-related fibrosis progression. *Am J Gastroenterol* 2002; **97**: 2408–14.

23. Poynter ME, Daynes RA. Peroxysome proliferator-activated receptor α activation modulates cellular redox status, represses nuclear factor-κB signaling, and reduces inflammatory cytokine production in aging. *J Biol Chem* 1998; **273**: 32833–41.

24. Pol S, Fontaine H, Carnot F, et al. Predictive factors for development of cirrhosis in parenterally acquired chronic hepatitis C: A comparison between immunocompetent and immunocompromised patients. *J Hepatol* 1998; **29**: 12–19.

25. Soriano V, Sulkowski M, Bergin C, et al. Care of patients with chronic hepatitis C and HIV co-infection: Recommendations from the HIV-HCV International Panel. *AIDS* 2002; **16**: 813–28.

26. Poynard T, Mathurin P, Lai CL, et al. A comparison of fibrosis progression in chronic liver diseases. *J Hepatol* 2003; **38**: 257–65.

27. De Moliner L, Pontisson P, De Salvo GL, et al. Serum and liver HCV RNA levels in patients with chronic hepatitis C: Correlation with clinical and histological features. *Gut* 1998; **42**: 856–60.

28. Roffi L, Ricci A, Ogliari CJ, et al. HCV genotypes in northern Italy: A survey of 1368 histologically proven chronic hepatitis C patients. *J Hepatol* 1998; **29**: 701–6.

29. Mathurin P, Moussalli J, Cadranel JF, et al. Slow progression rate of fibrosis in hepatitis C virus patients with persistently normal alanine transaminase activity. *Hepatology* 1998; **27**: 868–72.

30. Alberti A, Noventa F, Benvegnu L, Boccato S, Gatta A. Prevalence of liver disease in a population of asymptomatic persons with hepatitis C virus infection. Ann Intern Med 2002; **137**: 961–4.

31. Gumber SC, Chopra SC. Hepatitis C: A multifaced disease. Review to extrahepatic manifestations. *Ann Intern Med* 1995; **123**: 615–20.

32. Cacoub P, Poynard T, Ghillani P, et al., for the Multivirc Group. Extrahepatic manifestations in patients with chronic hepatitis C. *Arthritis Rheum* 1999; **42:** 2204–12.

33. El-Serag HB, Hampel H, Yeh C, Rabeneck L. Extrahepatic manifestations of hepatitis C among United States male veterans. *Hepatology* 2002; **36:** 1439–45.

34. El-Serag HB, Kunik M, Richardson P, Rabeneck L. Psychiatric disorders among veterans with hepatitis C infection. *Gastroenterology* 2002; **123:** 476–82.

35. Poynard T, Cacoub P, Ratziu V, et al. [Multivirc Group]. Fatigue in patients with chronic hepatitis C. *J Viral Hepat* 2002; **9:** 295–303.

36. Zuckerman E, Zuckerman T, Levine AM, et al. Hepatitis C virus infection in patients with B-cell non-Hodgkin lymphoma. *Ann Intern Med* 1997; **127:** 423–8.

37. Hermine O, Lefrere F, Bronowicki JP, et al. Regression of splenic lymphoma with lymphocytes after treatment of hepatitis C virus infection. *N Engl J Med* 2002; **347:** 89–94.

38. Marcellin P, Pouteau M, Benhamou JP. Hepatitis C virus infection, alpha interferon therapy and thyroid dysfunction. *J Hepatol* 1995; **22:** 364–9.

39. Foster GR, Goldin RD, Thomas HC. Chronic hepatitis C virus infection causes a significant reduction in quality of life in the absence of cirrhosis. *Hepatology* 1998; **27:** 209–12.

40. Rodger AJ, Jolley D, Thompson SC, Lanigan A, Crofts N. The impact of diagnosis of hepatitis C virus on quality of life. *Hepatology* 1999; **30:** 1299–301.

41. Bonkovsky HL, Woolley JM, and the Consensus Interferon Study Group. Reduction of health-related quality in chronic hepatitis C and improvement with interferon therapy. *Hepatology* 1999; **29:** 264–70.

42. Ware JE, Bayliss MS, Mannocchia M, Davis GL. Health-related quality of life in chronic hepatitis C: Impact of disease and treatment response. The Interventional Therapy Group. *Hepatology* 1999; **30:** 550–5.

43. Poynard T, Yuan MF, Ratziu V, Lai CL. Viral hepatitis C and B: Review. *Lancet* 2003; **362:** 2095–100.

44. Hickman IJ, Clouston AD, Macdonald GA, et al. Effect of weight reduction on liver histology and biochemistry in patients with chronic hepatitis C. *Gut* 2002; **51:** 89–94.

45. Thevenot T, Regimbeau C, Ratziu V, et al. Meta-analysis of interferon randomized trials in the treatment of viral hepatitis C in naive patients: 1999 update. *J Viral Hepat* 2001; **8:** 48–62.

46. Poynard T, Marcellin P, Lee S, et al. Randomised trial of interferon alpha 2b plus ribavirin for 48 weeks or for 24 weeks versus interferon alpha 2b plus placebo for 48 weeks for treatment of chronic infection with hepatitis C virus. *Lancet* 1998; **352:** 1426–32.

47. McHutchison JG, Gordon SC, Schiff ER, et al. Interferon alfa 2b alone or in combination with ribavirin as initial treatment for chronic hepatitis C. *N Engl J Med* 1998; **339:** 1485–92.

48. Poynard T, McHutchison J, Goodman Z, Ling MH, Albrecht J. Is an "à la carte" combination interferon alfa-2b plus ribavirin regimen possible for the first line treatment in patients with chronic hepatitis C? *Hepatology* 2000; **31:** 211–18.

49. Lindsay K, Trepo C, Heintges T, et al. A randomised, double-blind trial comparing pegylated interferon alfa-2b to interferon alfa-2b as initial treatment for chronic hepatitis C. *Hepatology* 2001; **34:** 395–403.

50. Zeuzem S, Feinman SV, Rasenack J, et al. Peginterferon alfa-2a in patients with chronic hepatitis C and cirrhosis. *N Engl J Med* 2000; **343:** 1673–80.

51. Heathcote EJ, Shiffman ML, Cooksley WGE, et al. Peginterferon alfa-2a in patients with chronic hepatitis C and cirrhosis. *N Engl J Med* 2000; **343:** 1673–80.

52. Manns MP, McHutchison JG, Gordon SC, et

al. PEG-interferon alfa-2b in combination with ribavirin compared to interferon alfa-2b plus ribavirin for initial treatment of chronic hepatitis C. *Lancet* 2001; **358**: 958–65.

53. Fried M, Shiffman ML, Reddy KR, et al. Peginterferon alfa-2a plus ribavirin for chronic hepatitis C virus infection. *N Engl J Med* 2002; **347**: 975–82.

54. Luise S, Bernardinello E, Calvetto L, et al. Kinetic of virological response during PEG-IFNs in chronic hepatitis C. *J Hepatol* 2004; **40**: 144 (abstract).

55. Hadziyannis SJ, Cheinquer H, Morgan T, et al. Peginterferon alfa-2a (40 kD) (PEGASYS) in combination with ribavirin (RBV): Efficacy and safety results from a phase III, randomised, double-blind, multicentre study examining effect of duration of treatment and RBV dose. *J Hepatol* 2002; **36** (Suppl 1): 3.

56. Poynard T, McHutchison J, Davis GL, et al. Impact of interferon alfa-2b and ribavirin on progression of liver fibrosis in patients with chronic hepatitis C. *Hepatology* 2000; **32**: 1131–7.

57. Poynard T, McHutchison J, Manns M, et al. Impact of pegylated interferon alfa-2b and ribavirin on liver fibrosis in patients with chronic hepatitis C. *Gastroenterology* 2002; **122**: 1303–13.

58. Cacoub P, Ratziu V, Myers RP, et al. [Multivirc Group]. Impact of treatment on extrahepatic manifestations in patients with chronic hepatitis C. *J Hepatol* 2002; **36**: 812–18.

59. Consensus Statement. EASL International Consensus Conference on Hepatitis C. *J Hepatol* 1999; **30**: 956–61.

60. Shiffman ML, Hofmann CM, Melissa J, et al. A randomized, controlled trial of maintenance interferon therapy for patients with chronic hepatitis C virus and persistent viremia. *Gastroenterology* 1999; **117**: 1164–72.

61. Glue P, Fang JW, Rouzier-Panis R, et al. Pegylated interferon-alfa2b: pharmacokinetics, pharmacodynamics, safety, and preliminary efficacy data. Hepatitis C Intervention Therapy Group. *Clin Pharmacol Ther* 2000; **68**: 556–67.

62. Zeuzem S, Hultcrantz R, Bourliere M, et al. Peginterferon alfa-2b plus ribavirin for treatment of chronic hepatitis C in previously untreated patients infected with HCV genotypes 2 or 3. *J Hepatol* 2004 (in press).

63. Algranati NE, Sy S, Modi M. A branched methoxy 40 kDa polyethylene glycol (PEG) moiety optimizes the pharmacokinetics (PK) of peginterferon (alpha)-2a (PEG-IFN) and may explain its enhanced efficacy in chronic hepatitis C (CHC) [Abstract]. *Hepatology* 1999; **30**: Suppl: 109A.

64. Poynard T, Ratzio V, McHutchison J, et al. Effect of treatment with peginterferon alfa-2b and ribavirin on steatosis in patients infected with hepatitis C. *Hepatology* 2003; **38**: 75–85.

65. Zeuzem S, Hultcrantz R, Bourliere M, et al. PEG-Interferon alfa-2b 1.5 μg/kg plus ribavirin 800–1400 mg/day for 24 weeks in patients with HCV2 or 3. *Hepatology* 2003; **38**: 1326.

66. McHutchison JG, Manns M, Patel K, et al. Adherence to combination therapy enhances sustained response in genotype-I-infected patients with chronic hepatitis C. *Gastroenterology* 2002; **123**: 1061–9.

67. Davis GL, Esteban-Mur R, Rustgi V, et al. Interferon alfa 2b alone or in combination with ribavirin for the treatment of relapse of chronic hepatitis C. *N Engl J Med* 1998; **339**: 1493–9.

68. Deuffic-Burban S, Poynard T, Valleron AJ. Quantification of fibrosis progression in patients with chronic hepatitis C using a Markov model. *J Viral Hepat* 2002; **9**: 114–22.

69. Shiratori Y, Imazeki F, Moriyama M, et al. Histological improvement of fibrosis in patients with hepatitis C who have sustained response to interferon therapy. *Ann Intern Med* 2000; **132**: 517–24.

70. Nishiguchi S, Kuroki T, Nakatani S, et al. Randomized trial of effects of interferon alfa on incidence of hepatocellular carcinoma in chronic active hepatitis C with cirrhosis. *Lancet* 1995; **346**: 1051–5.

71. Poynard T, Moussalli J, Ratziu V, et al. Is antiviral treatment (IFN alpha and/or ribavirin) justified in cirrhosis related to hepatitis C virus? Société Royale Belge de Gastroenterologie. *Acta Gastroenterol Belg* 1998; **61**: 431–7.

72. Yoshida H, Shiratori Y, Moriyama M, et al. Interferon therapy reduces the risk for hepatocellular carcinoma: national surveillance program of cirrhotic and noncirrhotic patients with chronic hepatitis C in Japan. *Ann Intern Med* 1999; **131**: 174–81.

73. Baffis V, Shrier I, Sherker AH, Szilagyi A. Use of interferon for prevention of hepatocellular carcinoma in cirrhotic patients with hepatitis B or hepatitis C virus infection. *Ann Intern Med* 1999; **131**: 696–701.

74. Yoshida H, Arakawa Y, Sata M, et al. Interferon therapy prolonged life expectancy among chronic hepatitis C patients. *Gastroenterology* 2002; **123**: 483–91.

75. Bruno S, Battezzati PM, Bellati G, et al. Long-term beneficial effects in sustained responders to interferon-alfa therapy for chronic hepatitis C. *J Hepatol* 2001; **34**: 748–55.

76. Camma C, Giunta M, Andreone P, Craxi A. Interferon and prevention of hepatocellular carcinoma in viral cirrhosis: an evidence-based approach. *J Hepatol* 2001; **34**: 593–602.

77. Schlam SW, Weiland O, Hansen BE, et al. Interferon-ribavirin for chronic hepatitis C with and without cirrhosis: analysis of individual patient data of six controlled trials. Eurohep Study Group for Viral Hepatitis. *Gastroenterology* 1999; **117**: 408–13.

78. Benhamou Y, Di Martino V, Bochet M, et al. Factors affecting liver fibrosis in human immunodeficiency virus- and hepatitis C virus-coinfected patients: impact of protease inhibitor therapy. *Hepatology* 2001; **34**: 283–7.

79. Zylberberg H, Benhamou Y, Lagneaux JL, et al. Safety and efficacy of interferon-ribavirin combination therapy of HCV-HIV coinfected subjects: an early report. *Gut* 2000; **47**: 694–7.

80. Gane EJ, Portmann BC, Naoumov NV, et al. Long-term outcome of hepatitis C infection after liver transplantation. *N Engl J Med* 1996; **334**: 815–20.

81. Berenguer M, Ferrell L, Watson J, et al. HCV-related fibrosis progression following liver transplantation: increase in recent years. *J Hepatol* 2000; **32**: 673–84.

82. Wali M, Harrison RF, Gow PJ, Mutimer D. Advancing donor liver age and rapid fibrosis progression following transplantation for hepatitis C. *Gut* 2002; **51**: 248–52.

83. Bizollon T, Palazzo U, Ducerf C, et al. Pilot study of the combination of interferon alfa and ribavirin as therapy of recurrent hepatitis C after liver transplantation. *Hepatology* 1997; **26**: 500–4.

84. Gane EJ, Lo SK, Riordan SM, et al. A randomized study comparing ribavirin and interferon alfa monotherapy for hepatitis C recurrence after liver transplantation. *Hepatology* 1998; **27**: 1403–7.

85. Samuel D, Bizollon T, Feray C, et al. Interferon-alpha 2b plus ribavirin in patients with chronic hepatitis C after liver transplantation: a randomized study. *Gastroenterology* 2003; **124**: 642–50.

86. Sheiner PA, Boros P, Klion FM, et al. The efficacy of prophylactic interferon alfa-2b in preventing recurrent hepatitis C after liver transplantation. *Hepatology* 1998; **28**: 831–8.

87. Mazzaferro V, Regalia E, Pulvirenti A, et al. Prophylaxis against HCV recurrence after liver transplantation: effect of interferon and ribavirin combination. *Transplant Proc* 1997; **29**: 519–21.

88. Neff GW, Bonham A, Tzakis AG, et al. Orthotopic liver transplantation in patients with human immunodeficiency virus and end-stage liver disease. *Liver Transpl* 2003; **9**: 239–47.

89. Fabrizi F, Poordad FF, Martin P. Hepatitis C infection and the patient with end-stage renal disease. *Hepatology* 2002; **36**: 3–10.

90. Bruchfeld A, Stahle L, Andersson J, Schvarcz R. Ribavirin treatment in dialysis patients

with chronic hepatitis C infection—a pilot study. *J Viral Hepat* 2001; **8**: 287–92.

91. Goedert JJ, Eyster ME, Lederman MM, et al. End-stage liver disease in persons with hemophilia and transfusion-associated infections. *Blood* 2002; **100**: 1584–9.

92. Ragni MV, Belle SH. Impact of human immunodeficiency virus infection on progression to end-stage liver disease in individuals with hemophilia and hepatitis C virus infection. *J Infect Dis* 2001; **183**: 1112–15.

93. Lesens O, Deschenes M, Steben M, Belanger G, Tsoukas CM. Hepatitis C virus is related to progressive liver disease in human immunodeficiency virus-positive hemophiliacs and should be treated as an opportunistic infection. *J Infect Dis* 1999; **179**: 1254–8.

94. Wilde J, Teixeira P, Bramhall SR, et al. Liver transplantation in haemophilia. *Br J Haematol* 2002; **117**: 952–6.

95. Lethagen S, Widell A, Berntorp E, Verbaan H, Lindgren S. Clinical spectrum of hepatitis C-related liver disease and response to treatment with interferon and ribavirin in haemophilia or von Willebrand's disease. *Br J Haematol* 2001; **113**: 87–93.

96. Venkataramani A, Behling C, Rond R, Glass C, Lyche K. Liver biopsies in adult hemophiliacs with hepatitis C: A United States center's experience. *Am J Gastroenterol* 2000; **95**: 2374–6.

97. Telfer P. Liver biopsy for haemophilic patients with chronic HCV infection. *Br J Haematol* 1997; **99**: 239–40.

98. Wong VS, Baglin T, Beacham E, et al. The role for liver biopsy in haemophiliacs infected with the hepatitis C virus. *Br J Haematol* 1997; **97**: 343–7.

99. Ahmed MM, Mutimer DJ, Elias E, et al. A combined management protocol for patients with coagulation disorders infected with hepatitis C virus. *Br J Haematol* 1996; **95**: 383–8.

100. Hanley JP, Jarvis LM, Andrews J, et al. Investigation of chronic hepatitis C infection in individuals with haemophilia: Assessment of invasive and non-invasive methods. *Br J Haematol* 1996; **94**: 159–65.

101. Prati D, Zanella A, Farma E, et al. A multicenter prospective study on the risk of acquiring liver disease in anti-hepatitis C virus negative patients affected from homozygous beta-thalassemia. *Blood* 1998; **92**: 3460–4.

102. Telfer PT, Garson JA, Whitby K, et al. Combination therapy with interferon alpha and ribavirin for chronic hepatitis C virus infection in thalassaemic patients. *Br J Haematol* 1997; **98**: 850–5.

103. Li CK, Chan PK, Ling SC, Ha SY. Interferon and ribavirin as frontline treatment for chronic hepatitis C infection in thalassaemia major. *Br J Haematol* 2002; **117**: 755–8.

104. Sievet W, Pianko S, Warner S, et al. Hepatic iron overload does not prevent a sustained virological response to interferon-alpha therapy: A long term follow-up study in hepatitis C-infected patients with beta thalassemia major. *Am J Gastroenterol* 2002; **97**: 982–7.

105. Sherker AH, Senosier M, Kermack D. Treatment of transfusion-dependent thalassemic patients infected with hepatitis C virus with interferon alpha-2b and ribavirin. *Hepatology* 2003; **37**: 223.

106. Giardini C, Galimberti M, Lucarelli G, et al. Alpha-interferon treatment of chronic hepatitis C after bone marrow transplantation for homozygous beta-thalassemia. *Bone Marrow Transplant* 1997; **20**: 767–72.

107. Talal AH, Weisz K, Hau T, Kreiswirth S, Dieterich DT. A preliminary study of erythropoietin for anemia associated with ribavirin and interferon-alpha. *Am J Gastroenterol* 2001; **96**: 2802–4.

108. Gergely AE, Lafarge P, Fouchard-Hubert I, Lunel-Fabiani F. Treatment of ribavirin/interferon-induced anemia with erythropoietin in patients with hepatitis C. *Hepatology* 2002; **35**: 1281–2.

109. Van Thiel DH, Faruki H, Friedlander L, et al. Combination treatment of advanced HCV

associated liver disease with interferon and G-CSF. *Hepatogastroenterology* 1995; **42**: 907–12.

110. Pardo M, Castillo I, Navas S, Carreno V. Treatment of chronic hepatitis C with cirrhosis with recombinant human granulocyte colony-stimulating factor plus recombinant interferon-alpha. *J Med Virol* 1995; **45**: 439–44.

111. Artz AS, Ershler WB, Rustgi V. Interleukin-11 for thrombocytopenia associated with hepatitis C. *J Clin Gastroenterol* 2001; **33**: 425–6.

112. Fried MW. Side effects of therapy of hepatitis C and their management. *Hepatology* 2002; **36** (5 Suppl 1): S237–44.

113. Wong JB, Bennett WG, Koff RS, Pauker SG. Pretreatment evaluation of chronic hepatitis C: Risks, benefits, and costs. *JAMA* 1998; **280**: 2088–93.

114. Younossi ZM, Singer ME, McHutchison JG, Shermock KM. Cost effectiveness of interferon 2b combined with ribavirin for the treatment of chronic hepatitis C. *Hepatology* 1999; **30**: 1318–24.

115. Wong JB, Poynard T, Ling MH, Albrecht JK, Pauker SG. Cost-effectiveness of 24 or 48 weeks of interferon alpha-2b alone or with ribavirin as initial treatment of chronic hepatitis C. International Hepatitis Interventional Therapy Group. *Am J Gastroenterol* 2000; **95**: 1524–30.

116. Siebert U, Sroczynski G, Rossol S, et al. Cost effectiveness of peginterferon alpha-2b plus ribavirin versus interferon alpha-2b plus ribavirin for initial treatment of chronic hepatitis C. *Gut* 2003; **52**: 425–32.

117. Wright TL, Cooper S. Acute hepatitis C. *Hepatology* 2001; **33**: 321–7.

118. Villano SA, Vlahov D, Nelson KE, Cohn S, Thomas DL. Persistence of viremia and the importance of long-term follow-up after acute hepatitis C infection. *Hepatology* 1999; **29**: 908–14.

119. Giuberti T, Marin MG, Ferrari C, et al. Hepatitis C virus viremia following clinical resolution of acute hepatitis C. *J Hepatol* 1994; **20**: 666–71.

120. Poynard T, Regimbeau C, Myers RP, et al. Interferon for acute hepatitis C. Cochrane Review. *Cochrane Database Syst Rev* 2002; 1.

121. Jaeckel E, Cornberg M, Wedemeyer H, et al. Treatment of acute hepatitis C with interferon alfa-2b. *N Engl J Med* 2001; **345**: 1452–7.

122. Poynard T, Ratziu V, Bedossa P. Appropriateness of liver biopsy. *Can J Gastroenterol* 2000; **14**: 543–8.

123. Imbert-Bismut F, Ratziu V, Pieroni L, et al. Biochemical markers of liver fibrosis in patients with hepatitis C virus infection: A prospective study. *Lancet* 2001; **357**: 1069–75.

124. Pawlotsky JM, Bouvier-Alias M, Hezode C, et al. Standardization of hepatitis C virus RNA quantification. *Hepatology* 2000; **32**: 654–9.

125. Bouvier-Alias M, Patel K, Dahari H, et al. Clinical utility of total HCV core antigen quantification: a new indirect marker of HCV replication. *Hepatology* 2002; **36**: 211–18.

126. Hinrichsen H, Benhamou Y, Reiser M, et al. First report on the antiviral efficacy of BILN 2061, a novel oral HCV serine protease inhibitor, in patients with chronic hepatitis C genotype 1 [Abstract]. *Hepatology* 2002; **36**: 379A.

127. Benhamou Y, Hinrichsen H, Sentjens R, et al. Safety, tolerability and antiviral effect of BILN 2061, a novel HCV serine protease inhibitor, after oral treatment over 2 days in patients with chronic hepatitis C, genotype 1, with advanced liver fibrosis [Abstract]. *Hepatology* 2002; **36**: 304A.

128. Lamarre D, Anderson PC, Bailey M, et al. An N53 protease inhibitor with antiviral effects in humans infected with hepatitis C virus. *Nature* 2003; **426**: 186–9.

129. Forns X, Bukh J, Purcell RH. The challenge of developing a vaccine against hepatitis C virus. *J Hepatol* 2002; **37**: 684–95.

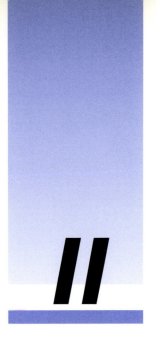

Hepatitis B

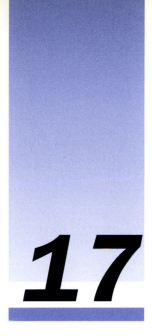

Natural history of hepatitis B: Epidemiology

Despite the discovery of the virus more than 30 years ago,[1] the efficacy of hepatitis B (HBV) vaccine[2] and the advances in therapy (Figure 17.1), hepatitis B still remains an important public health problem (Table 17.1).

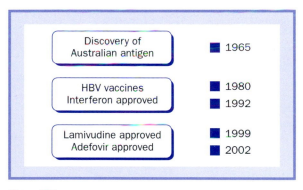

Figure 17.1
Landmarks in hepatitis B.

Prevalence

According to the World Health Organization (WHO), one-third of the world's population (2 billion people) have been infected with HBV, and about 5% are chronically infected (more than 350 000 million people).[2,3]

These individuals are at risk of developing hepatologic and nonhepatologic manifestations. Between one-third and one-quarter of people infected chronically with HBV are expected to develop progressive liver disease (including cirrhosis and

Table 17.1 Risk groups for HBV infection among nonvaccinated people.

Areas of high HBV prevalence	*Vertical transmission: infants born to HBV-infected mothers* *Horizontal transmission within families (first 10 years)*
Areas of intermediate HBV prevalence	*Horizontal transmission: older children, adolescents and adults*
Areas of low prevalence	*High-risk sexual behavior, multiple partners, HIV, genital herpes* *Injection drug users even briefly many years ago* *Frequent exposure to blood products: hemophilia, transplants, hemodialysis, chronic renal failure, gamma globulins, cancer chemotherapy* *Health-care workers with needle-stick accidents* *Blood transfusion before 1970*

primary liver cancer). Hepatitis B can cause cirrhosis, digestive hemorrhage, liver failure and liver cancer.[2,3]

Serologic markers and interpretation

The knowledge of the virus genome has permitted us to have several serologic markers of HBV infection.[4] Hepatitis B surface antigen (HBsAg), HBeAg and anti-HBe are tested by the enzyme-linked immunoabsorbent assay (ELISA). The presence of HBsAg in the serum for 6 months or more is indicative of chronic hepatitis B infection. The estimated annual incidence for clearance of HBsAg in chronically infected patients is low (0.1–0.8%) and is usually due to a decrease in viremia rather than the emergence of HBsAg mutants.[5]

Commonly used commercial assays for HBV-DNA levels are the branched DNA (bDNA) assay and the hybrid capture test.[4] The lower limits of detection for these two assays are 700 000 and 140 000 copies/mL, respectively. One commercially available PCR assay allows the detection of 200 copies/mL. The interpretation of HBV serologic markers is described in Table 18.1.

In clinical practice, chronic HBV carriers may be divided into two easily identifiable serologic types: those who are positive for HBeAg ("wild-type") and those who are HBeAg negative and positive for anti-HBe.

HBV variants

The repression of the synthesis of the wild-type HBV is due to defective variants with mutation in the core region. Among these variants, the most common in the Mediterranean area is a mutant containing a strategic mutation at nucleotide 1896 of the precore region that prevents the secretion of

HBeAg ("precore mutant").[6-9] HBeAg-negative, anti-HBe-positive chronic hepatitis B accounts for 7–30% of patients with chronic hepatitis worldwide. Prevalence rates range from 40–80% in the Mediterranean area, Hong Kong, Korea, Taiwan and Japan to 13–15% in India and China, and lower rates in northern Europe and the USA. The geographic variability in the prevalence of precore mutants may be related to the geographic variability of the HBV genotype.

Most variants seem to occur in the long-term natural history of wild-type HBV, but the exact prevalence of direct infection (transfusion, vertical or sexual) is unknown.[8-11] Several studies have documented progression from wild-type to mutation 1896.[9,10]

HBV genotypes

Full-length sequence and phylogenetic analysis have isolated eight genotypes from A to H, the most prevalent in Western countries being genotypes A and D.[9-11] Subtypes are the variation of amino acids on the HBsAg. The standard four are adr, adw, ayw and ayr. The most frequent combinations of the genotypes and subtypes are genotypes A (subtype adw) in Western Europe, D (subtype ayw) in the Mediterranean area and G in France.

Genotypes D and F of HBV tolerate the 1896 mutation, whereas the mutation occurring within A and E genotypes generates nonviable mutants. The prevalence of genotype D matches the prevalence of precore mutants in the Mediterranean area. Mutation 1896 seems more frequent in genotype D than in genotype A.

Routes of transmission

The predominant routes of transmission vary according to the endemicity of the HBV infection. In areas of high endemicity, perinatal transmission is the main route of transmission, whereas in areas of low endemicity, sexual contact among high-risk adults is predominant.[9-12]

Most of the "transmission" of *chronic* HBV infection is perinatal transmission. For neonates and children under the age of 1 year who acquire the infection, the risk of chronicity is 90%. For children 1–5 years of age, the risk is approximately 30%. For children over 5 years old and for adults, the risk from pooled data decreases to around 2%. The reason(s) for the high risk of chronicity in neonates and in children under the age of 1 year is still uncertain. It has been postulated that transplacental passage of the hepatitis B e antigen (HBeAg) from an infected mother to the fetus may induce immunologic tolerance of the virus. However, a study in transgenic mice shows that the placenta is an efficient barrier to HBeAg transfer.[13]

Because of the age-related risk of chronicity, the predominant sources of transmission for persons who become chronically infected are infected mothers at birth or in the postnatal period, and less commonly, infected fathers, siblings and relatives, through close contact during early childhood.

Sexual contact, intravenous drug use and acupuncture can also transmit the disease. Transfusion-related hepatitis B is rare, since screening for hepatitis B has been a routine in transfusion centers for at least two decades. For all these latter modes of transmission, the risk of chronicity is low.

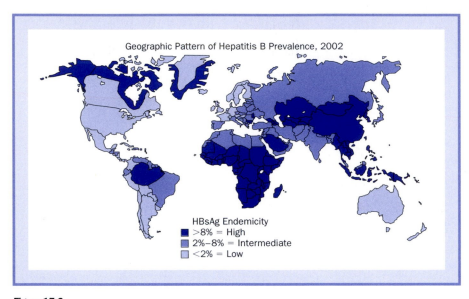

Figure 17.2
Worldwide prevalence of HBV.
Source: WHO weekly epidemiology record, No. 6, 2002, **77,** *41–48.*

Three-quarters of the world's chronic hepatitis B subjects are Chinese. The other area of high endemicity of chronic hepatitis B is sub-Saharan Africa and the western Pacific. The prevalence of chronic hepatitis B in these areas is 10–20%, with the majority of infection occurring at the neonate period, or early childhood. In contrast, the prevalence is low (0.2–0.5%) in North America, northern, western and central Europe, and Australia, where the majority of infection occurs during adolescence or adulthood through sexual contact or intravenous drug use (Figure 17.2).

Natural history of hepatitis B: Hepatic manifestations

The major hepatologic consequence is the progression to cirrhosis and its potential complications: hemorrhage, hepatic insufficiency and primary liver cancer[9–12] (Table 18.2).

Unlike HCV infection, current understanding of the natural history of HBV infection has not been well analyzed by assessment of liver fibrosis progression.[14–18] The three classical phases of chronic hepatitis B disease have been described without many histologic studies: (1) a prolonged immune tolerance phase in childhood and adolescents with near normal histology, high HBV-DNA levels and HBeAg positivity; (2) the immune clearance phase with seroconversion from HBeAg to antibody against HBeAg (anti-HBe) accompanied by active inflammation and fibrosis, and fluctuating serum alanine transaminase (ALT) levels; (3) the residual phase with low HBV-DNA and normal ALT levels.

Age at infection, persistence and strength of replication, virus genotype, emergence of viral mutants and integration of viral genomic material into the hepatocyte genome play a role in the natural history. So far, the relationships of these factors to fibrosis progression have not been clearly assessed.

Age at infection

The age at infection is most often unknown in patients without vertical transmission, a condition which does not facilitate modeling of fibrosis progression.[18] The age at infection affects the course of the disease. For those who

Table 18.1 Interpretation of serologic markers according to symptoms, transaminases and histologic features.

	HBsAg	HBsAb	HBeAg	HBeAb	Anti-HBc-IgG	Anti-HBc-IgM	HBV DNA	Symptoms	ALT	Histologic activity and fibrosis
Acute	+	−	+	±	+	+	+	±	++	+
Chronic carrier wild-type	+	−	+	−	+	−	+	±	±	+
Chronic carrier precore mutant[1]	+	−	−	+	+	±	+	±	±	+
"Healthy carrier"[2]	+	−	−	−	+	−	−	−	−	−
"Immune tolerance"[2]	+	−	+	−	+	−	++	−	−	−
Recovery/immunity	−	+	−	+	+	−	−	−	−	−
Immunity from vaccination	−	+	−	−	−	−	−	−	−	−
Occult infection[3]	−	±	−	−	±	−	±	±	±	±

[1]During flare-up, anti-HBc-IgM may be elevated.
[2]Carriers without symptoms, with normal transaminases and with normal biopsy are divided into "healthy carriers" with undetectable HBV DNA and subjects with detectable HBV DNA ("Immune tolerance"). In these patients, a risk of cirrhosis or hepatocellular carcinoma cannot be excluded. Precore mutant can be detected.
[3]HBV DNA can be detected in the liver in absence of serologic markers.

Table 18.2 Natural history of HBV carriers.

First author	Number	Age at baseline	Duration of follow-up	Evolution	Liver complications	Death related to liver
Bortolotti HbeAg-positive baseline HbeAg-negative baseline	185 168 17	<10 years	13 years	5% became HBsAg negative 7% still HBe positive 83% became anti-HBe and asymptomatic 3% reactivation 2% elevated transaminases and anti-HBe	2 hepatocellular carcinoma	
MacMahon	1400	46 years	5 years	No vasculitis or cryoglobulinemia	14 chronic active hepatitis 8 cirrhosis 20 hepatocellular carcinoma	13 hepatocellular carcinoma
Sakuma	202	45 years	5 years	9% persistent abnormal transaminases 76% persistent normal transaminases	5 hepatocellular carcinoma (4 cirrhosis)	4 hepatocellular carcinoma (3 had normal transaminases at baseline)

acquire the disease during adolescence or adulthood (the majority of the Caucasian population), there is no immune tolerance phase. Instead, the disease progresses directly to the immune clearance phase and is of relatively short duration. This could explain why the Caucasian patients with HBeAg seroconversion and low HBV-DNA levels do not have progressive disease, becoming "healthy carriers".[19] In contrast, for those who acquire the disease during the neonatal period and early childhood (the majority of the Asian and African population), the disease continues to progress in a proportion of patients after HBeAg seroconversion.[12]

Persistence and strength of replication

The sensitivity of HBV-DNA assays is improving every year, and therefore is changing the definition of replicative stages.[4]

In general, HBV is not a cytopathic virus. In most patients with chronic hepatitis B, there is no direct correlation between the serum viral load and the severity of liver disease. A level of less than 10^5 copies/mL has been suggested to be associated with HBeAg seroconversion and inactive disease,[20] but this is still controversial.[21]

Clinical signification of HBV variants

Few cross-sectional or longitudinal studies have compared the clinical significance of chronic HBV carriers who are positive for HBeAg ("wild-type") and those who are HBeAg negative and positive for anti-HBe[8,17,18] (Table 18.3). HBeAg-negative

patients were older, and this may explain the higher prevalence of significant fibrosis.[18]

Very few patients have been followed longitudinally with virologic assessment.[14–17] Among 12 HBeAg-positive patients with chronic hepatitis who seroconverted to anti-HBe during follow-up, anti-HBe seroconversion was accompanied by a dramatic reduction of hepatitis B virus replication and normalization of transaminases in all except one, and by the emergence of a precore mutant (1896 point mutation) that replaced the wild-type in seven of the 12. Of the seven who harbored the precore mutant, three continued to show normal transaminases during subsequent follow-up, three had mild transaminase elevation and one had an acute short-lived reactivation after 4 years of normal transaminases. The five patients who continued to show prevalence of wild-type in spite of anti-HBe seroconversion all revealed persistently normal transaminases.

Asians who are HBeAg negative have lower HBV-DNA levels than HBeAg-positive patients, but they continue to have exacerbations. There is no single cutoff HBV-DNA value to determine whether anti-HBe-positive patients will have inactive disease or continue to have exacerbations.[21] Severe exacerbations occur with equal frequency in HbeAg-positive and anti-Hbe-positive patients.[22]

Modeling is also complicated by the fact that precore mutations, formerly thought to be responsible for viral replication and disease activity after HBeAg seroconversion, are detected in up to 44% of HBeAg-positive patients. Disease activity after HBeAg seroconversion is not associated with precore

Table 18.3 Comparison between HBV carriers HBeAg positive versus anti-HBe positive.

First author	Number	Age (years) at biopsy	Male	Asian or African origin	HBV DNA detectable	Normal transaminases	Significant fibrosis (F2/F3/F4)	Cirrhosis	Significant activity (A2/A3)
Poynard									
HBeAg positive	491	35	74%	62%	100%	14%	22%	7%	50%
HBeAg negative	286	41	76%	43%	39%	43%	42%	15%	23%
HBV-DNApos	113	44	80%	17%	100%	11%	57%	21%	43%
HBV-DNAneg	173	40	73%	79%	0%	54%	32%	11%	19%
Zarski									
HBeAg positive	215	36	83%	17%	100%	100%		17%	
HBeAg negative	61	44	84%	26%	100%	100%		38%	

and core promoter mutations.[23] Two-thirds of cirrhosis-related complications and hepatocellular carcinoma in Asian hepatitis B patients occur after HBeAg seroconversion.[24]

Genotype

Caucasian patients with genotype A, compared to patients with genotype D, have a higher chance of clearance of HBV DNA and HBsAg, and sustained remission after HBeAg seroconversion, as well as lower necroinflammatory stages in liver biopsies.[25] Asian patients with genotype B, compared to patients with genotype C, have HBeAg seroconversion at an earlier age, comparatively less serious liver disease, and better response to interferon.[25–28] However, whether there is any difference between patients with genotypes B and C in development of hepatocellular carcinoma is still controversial.[29–31]

Can a healthy carrier state be defined?

Most longitudinal or cross-sectional studies in HBV have distinguished a "healthy" carrier state, a phase of chronic hepatitis and cirrhosis. The definition of "healthy HBV carrier" is not clear and therefore could be dangerous for patients. If the definition is the absence of symptoms, the absence of transaminase elevation and the absence of abnormalities in the liver (inflammation, necrosis or fibrosis), these negative findings should have been observed at least twice. This is not the case in the published cohorts. Despite an overall good prognosis,[32–35] the status of "healthy HBV carrier" is not definitive, and some patients may progress to cirrhosis and/or hepatocellular carcinoma[32,33] (Table 18.4). We observed significant fibrosis (septal fibrosis or cirrhosis) in 30% of 163 HBsAg-positive patients with undetectable serum HBV DNA.[35] Even in patients with the absence of hepatitis B surface antigen (HBsAg) and the presence of anti-HBs, liver complications may occur.[36]

Association with hepatocellular carcinoma

An association between HBV infection and the occurrence of primary liver cancer (hepatocellular carcinoma) was observed soon after the discovery of HBV and was largely confirmed thereafter.[37–39]

These lines of evidence were based on epidemiologic associations in areas of high prevalence,[37] on molecular studies in hepatocellular carcinoma cell lines,[40] and on animal models.[41] In endemic areas such as China and sub-Saharan Africa, where the HBsAg carrier rate is 10%, primary liver cancer presents an incidence of up to 150 cases per 100 000 per year. In contrast, in the United States where the carrier rate is less than 1%, the incidence of primary liver cancer is 4 cases per 100 000 per year. The prevalence of HBsAg among patients with primary liver cancer varies from 85–95% in Africa and Asia to 10–25% in Western Europe and the United States.[42] A further support for this association was the decrease in childhood primary liver cancer after implementation of universal vaccination of newborns.[43] The incidence of liver cancer among HBV carriers is associated with the duration of infection, male gender, and the age and the severity of liver disease[44] (Figure 18.1).

Table 18.4 *Natural history of "healthy carriers".*

First author	Number	Age at follow-up	Duration of follow-up	Liver complications	Death related to liver	HBsAg negativation rate per year
Villeneuve	317	46 years	16 years	0 liver cancer	4 cirrhosis	0.7%
De Franchis	92		10 years	1 cirrhosis 0 liver cancer	0	1%

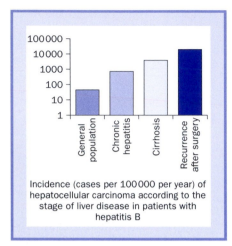

Figure 18.1
Annual incidence of hepatocellular carcinoma according to the stage of liver disease. Adapted with permission.[44]

Occult infection

HBV DNA can be detected in the liver of patients without detectable HBsAg in the serum.[45] The lack of HBsAg may be due to rearrangements in the HBV genome that interfere with gene expression or lead to the production of an antigenetically modified S protein.[46] Clearance of serum HBsAg may also occur without clearance of HBV DNA in the liver.[47]

Factors associated with fibrosis progression

There is little information concerning the annual rate of development of cirrhosis in chronic HBV carriers or of risk factors

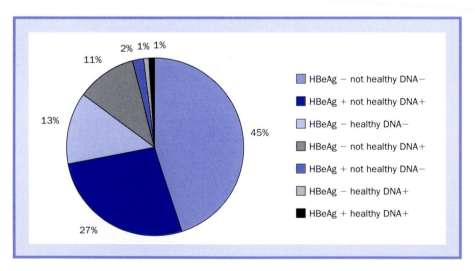

Figure 18.2
Prevalence of HBeAg and detectable HBV DNA in a cohort of 223 HBsAg-positive subjects. 70% of subjects were HBeAg negative. 15% of subjects were healthy carriers: absence of symptoms, normal transaminases, and absence of necrosis, inflammation and fibrosis at liver biopsy (A0F0). Among these healthy carriers, only four had detectable HBV DNA.

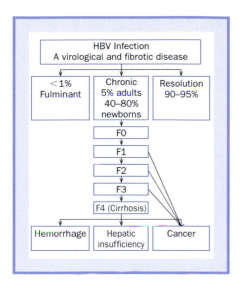

associated with the fibrosis progression rate. Factors associated and not associated with cirrhosis or hepatocellular carcinoma are summarized in Table 18.5.[3,7,8]

Figure 18.3
Natural history of hepatitis B virus infection. Estimated key numbers of HBV natural history from literature and our database. The median time from infection (F0) to cirrhosis (F4) is 30 years. The mortality rate at 10 years for cirrhosis is 50%. The transition probability per year from noncomplicated cirrhosis to each of the complications is around 3%. Less than 10% of cancer occurred in noncirrhotic liver.

Table 18.5 Factors associated with progression to cirrhosis or to cancer in HBV carriers.

Factors	Cirrhosis	Hepatocellular carcinoma
Age at infection	Yes	Yes
Duration of infection	Yes	Yes
Male gender	Yes	Yes
Age at biopsy	Yes	Yes
Consumption of alcohol >50 g per day	Yes	Yes
HCV coinfection	Yes	Not sure
Delta virus coinfection	Yes	Not sure
CD4 count <200/mL	Yes	Not sure
Fibrosis stage	Yes	Yes
Necrosis	Not sure	Not sure
Inflammation	Not sure	Not sure
Genotype	Not sure	Not sure
Precore mutant	Not sure	Not sure
Core-promoter mutant	Not sure	Not sure
Seroconversion anti-Hbe	Not sure	Not sure
HBV-DNA level	Not sure	Not sure
Aflatoxin	Not sure	Yes

Natural history of hepatitis B: Extrahepatic manifestations and quality of life

19

Extrahepatic manifestations

Since the recognition of the HBV virus, numerous extrahepatic manifestations have been reported with hepatitis B virus infection, including vasculitis (polyarteritis nodosa), glomerulonephritis, mixed cryoglobulinemia, skin rash, arthritis, arthralgia and papular acrodermatitis[48-55] (Table 19.1).

Table 19.1 Extrahepatic manifestations in HBV.

> **Chronic hepatitis**
> Polyarteritis nodosa
> Glomerulonephritis
>   Membranous
>   Mesangial proliferative
>   Membranoproliferative
> Cryoglobulinemia
>
> **Acute hepatitis**
> Arthralgia
> Arthritis
> Skin rashes
> Serum sickness-like manifestations
> Urticaria
> Papular acrodermatitis

Vasculitis

Systemic vasculitis (systemic necrotizing vasculitis or polyarteritis nodosa [PAN]) is the most severe symptomatic extrahepatic manifestation, although it is rare (1%). As many as 30–70% of patients with PAN are infected with HBV. The initial illness presents with abdominal pain, fever, rash, polyarthralgias, polyarthritis, hypertension and eosinophilia; it can progress to multisystem vasculitis involving the kidneys, gastrointestinal tract, and peripheral and central nervous systems. Medium to small arteries are involved by fibrinoid necrosis and perivascular infiltration. Angiographic findings include microaneurysms, stenosis and occlusion of arteries, mainly in the kidneys, the liver and the intestine. The mortality rate is high (30–50%) and is not associated with the hepatitis severity.

Glomerulonephritis

Most patients have the nephrotic syndrome, with 85% rate of spontaneous remission by 2 years. Despite the limited number of studies, the benign natural history seems to be more frequent in children than in adults. Membranous glomerulonephritis is the most common pathologic finding, especially in children, and is usually associated with capillary wall deposits of HBeAg. Membrano-proliferative glomerulonephritis is less frequent, most often described in adults and associated with capillary wall deposits of HBsAg. This form of glomerulonephritis seems to result from immune complex-mediated injury, but factors explaining why only a few patients experience this injury are unknown.[54]

Cryoglobulin

The strong association observed between mixed cryoglobulinemia and chronic hepatitis B was in retrospect mostly related to hepatitis C coinfection.[55] The prevalence of cryoglobulin-positive patients in hepatitis B is three times lower than in hepatitis C.

Cryoglobulin-positive patients have mixed type II cryoglobulins or type III.

Health-related quality of life

One way to assess the clinical impact of hepatic and extrahepatic manifestations among patients infected by HBV is to assess the health-related quality of life. Patients with chronic HBV infection showed a reduction in the SF36 scores that assessed mental functions, but they had no decrease in the scores that measured physical symptoms.[56,57]

Median utilities for mildly symptomatic HBV infection and severely symptomatic HBV infection are significantly decreased in comparison with asymptomatic HBV infection. For severely symptomatic HBV infection, there was no difference in comparison with the quality of life of patients with AIDS[57] (Figure 19.1).

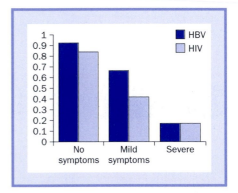

Figure 19.1
Quality of life is impaired among patients infected with hepatitis B. On a scale in which 0 was equivalent to death, and 1 was equivalent to good health, the median utilities were estimated by 200 house staff and staff physicians infected by HBV or HIV according to three stages. For HIV, severe infection was AIDS. All differences versus asymptomatic stage were significant (p < 0.01 or each two-way comparison). There was no difference between the two severe stages. Adapted with permission.[57]

Goal of treatment in chronic hepatitis B

20

The optimal goal of treatment is to eliminate the virus completely and permanently.[58] In fact, as in hepatitis C, there are now two separate goals: the first goal is to achieve a sustained clearance of the virus; the second goal in patients without a sustained virologic response is to reduce the liver injury, reduce fibrosis progression in noncirrhotic patients,[18] prevent cirrhosis complications, improve quality of life and reduce infectivity[59] (Table 20.1).

The arrival of nucleoside analog therapy marks a new era in the treatment of chronic hepatitis B. In the majority of clinical trials, the standard therapeutic endpoints have been virologic endpoints; the loss of HBeAg (with or without

Table 20.1 Endpoints of treatment in chronic hepatitis B.

Endpoints	Optimal goal	Suppressive goal
Seroconversion in HBsAg	Yes	No
Seroconversion in HBeAg for wild-type	Yes	No
Serum HBV DNA undetectable*	Yes	No
Normalization of transaminase activity	Yes	No
Disappearance of liver fibrosis	Yes	No
Disappearance of necrosis and inflammation	Yes	No
Reduction of fibrosis progression	Yes	Yes
Reduction of necrosis and inflammation	Yes	Yes
Improvement of quality of life	Yes	Yes
Reduction of infectivity	Yes	Yes
Reduction of morbidity	Yes	Yes
Reduction of mortality	Yes	Yes

*HBV-DNA detection methods have a large range of sensitivity from 2 (PCR assay) to 1 million copies/mL

anti-HBe positivity), together with undetectable HBV DNA as measured by bDNA or hybrid capture assays. From a regulatory perspective, several official agencies require and use histology as the principal endpoint. The total eradication of the virus is hardly ever achieved and is rarely used as a clinical trial or therapeutic endpoint.

However, with the knowledge that disease activity can continue with relatively low viral titers, and with the availability of more potent nucleoside analogs for clinical trials, HBV-DNA levels as measured by PCR assays are already being used as primary endpoints. The effect of the newer agents on HBV-DNA levels in liver biopsies is also being investigated, as well as the utility of biochemical markers.[60]

The arrival of nucleoside analog therapy has also facilitated the efficacy of transplantation, which must be discussed in nonresponders.

Efficacy of interferon and pegylated interferon (PEG-IFN)

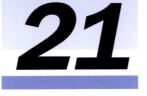

Biological effect

Interferon alfa was the first drug approved for the treatment of chronic hepatitis B in 1992 in the USA and Europe. Interferon alfa binds to specific cell receptors and produces immunomodulatory, antiviral and antifibrotic effects (Table 21.1). Interferon increases the activity of macrophages, natural killer cells and cytotoxic T cells, which mediate the elimination of virus-infected cells. Antiviral properties of interferon alfa include inhibition of virus entry into cells and the reduction of viral RNA and protein synthesis.

Table 21.1 Different effects of interferon alfa.

Antiviral effect	Immunomodulatory	Antifibrotic
Increases macrophage activity	Increases Th1 effect (IL-12)	Reduces stellate cell activation
Increases natural killer cell activity	Increases HLA I expression	Activates collagenases
Increase cytotoxic T-cell activity	Increases B-cell proliferation	
Activates 2-5-oligoadenylate synthetase which reduces viral RNA	Modulates Th2 effect	
Activates protein kinase P1, which reduces viral protein synthesis		

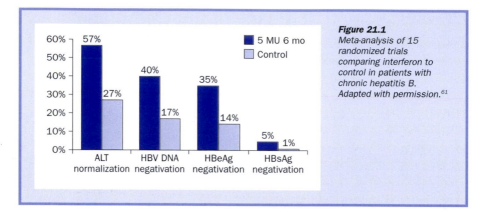

Figure 21.1
Meta-analysis of 15 randomized trials comparing interferon to control in patients with chronic hepatitis B. Adapted with permission.[61]

Clinical effect

Interferon alfa in doses of at least 5 million units three times a week has been shown to induce virologic and biological responses in 30–50% of treated patients in comparison with spontaneous remission rate of 5–15% in controls.[58,59,61] The recommended regimen of interferon alfa is either 5 million units daily or 10 million units thrice weekly, subcutaneously for 4 months.[58] Liver biopsy performed 6 months or more after completion of treatment demonstrates improvement in necrosis and inflammation.[62] Extrahepatic manifestations of infection have also demonstrated a response to interferon.[49]

Durability of response and long-term outcome

Interferon alfa-induced HBeAg clearance has been reported to be durable in 80–90% of patients after a follow-up period of 4–8 years.[58] Data on the long-term outcome of interferon-treated patients are limited. Patients who cleared HBeAg had better survival and survival free of hepatic decompensation[63] (Figures 21.2 and 21.3).

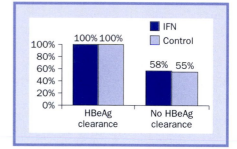

Figure 21.2
Long-term efficacy of interferon (IFN): 8-year survival and HBeAg status. Adapted with permission.[63]

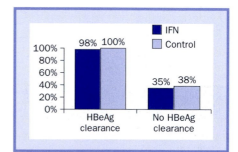

Figure 21.3
Long-term efficacy of interferon: 8-year survival without complications and HBeAg status. Adapted with permission.[63]

Predictive factors of response

Six factors are associated with a sustained beneficial response to interferon (Table 21.2). The most important are age, high transaminases and low serum HBV DNA. The response rates to interferon may vary greatly between Asian and Caucasian patients and only be similar when adjusted for age at infection, transaminases and HBV DNA.

Asian patients HBeAg positive, HBV DNA positive and persistently normal in ALT are usually children or young adults with perinatally acquired HBV infection. The response rate of interferon is lower than 10%, and the benefit-risk ratio is not known.

Up to 65% of Caucasian chronic hepatitis B patients who have HBeAg seroconversion will eventually also lose HBsAg. HBV DNA is usually still detectable after HBeAg seroconversion if the patients remain positive for HBsAg, but will become undetectable by PCR in 60–100% of those who lose HBsAg. Patients who have HBeAg seroconversion have a lower risk of developing hepatitis B cirrhosis-related complications than those who

remain positive for HBeAg. In addition, they have longer survival rates and longer intervals free from clinical complications.

There are two long-term follow-up studies for interferon alfa in the Asian population. In the Taiwan study of patients whose median ALT on entry into the study was >200 IU/L, there was a marginally significant increase in cumulative HBeAg seroconversion in the interferon alfa-treated groups.[64] There was significantly more hepatocellular carcinoma (HCC) in the untreated patients, but no difference, in the development of new cirrhosis and of cirrhosis with complications, between treated and untreated patients. In the second study from Hong Kong, the cumulative HBeAg seroconversion was similar in both the interferon alfa-treated and the untreated patients, irrespective of the ALT levels.[65] Complications of cirrhosis and HCC occurred with equal frequency in both groups. Some of the differences in the two studies are probably related to the fact that the patients in the Taiwan study had very active disease with fairly high ALT levels on entry into the trial.[59]

The long-term benefit of interferon in terms of reduction of fibrosis progression has not been evaluated.

In patients with compensated cirrhosis, interferon is safe and may be effective. In patients with decompensated cirrhosis, interferon is not contraindicated, but sepsis and exacerbation of liver disease have been described.[66]

Table 21.2 Factors associated with sustained beneficial response to interferon alfa in patients with chronic hepatitis B.

Favorable factors
Short duration of disease
Infection at adult age
High serum transaminase activity
Low serum HBV-DNA level
Active histologic changes (inflammation and necrosis)
Wild-type (HBeAg-positive) virus
Absence of decompensated cirrhosis
Absence of immunosuppression

Efficacy of PEG-IFN

In a preliminary trial, PEG-IFN alfa-2a had a more rapid, a greater decline in HBV DNA, and higher HBeAg seroconversion rate than standard interferon.[67]

Regimens using PEG-IFN alfa-2b for one year lead to sustained response in 44% of patients.[68]

Efficacy of lamivudine

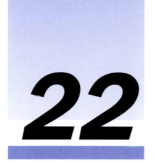

Lamivudine is the (−) enantiomer of 2',3'-dideoxy-3'-thiacytidine. It is phosphorylated to the triphosphate, which competes with the other triphosphates for incorporation into DNA, causing chain termination. By decreasing the viral load, lamivudine may also reverse the T-cell hyporesponsiveness to hepatitis B viral antigens.

Efficacy was observed first among patients coinfected by HIV and HBV.[68] Thereafter, several randomized clinical trials have demonstrated the efficacy of lamivudine 100 mg per day in immunocomponent patients infected by wild-type[70–72] or precore[73] HBV.

Efficacy in patients infected with wild-type HBV (HBeAg positive)

During 52 weeks of treatment, lamivudine was effective in comparison with placebo on almost all endpoints: transaminases, HBV DNA measured by non-PCR methods, HBe seroconversion, necrosis, inflammation and fibrosis. There was no difference for HBsAg. Long-term study has confirmed the efficacy of lamivudine on histologic features.[74]

Efficacy in patients infected with precore mutant HBV (HBeAg negative)

There are fewer trials in precore HBV infection. In one randomized trial, lamivudine was effective at 24 weeks versus placebo[73] on transaminases and HBV DNA (Figure 22.4).

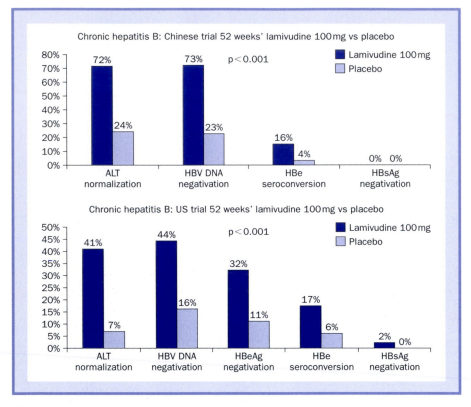

Figure 22.1
Efficacy of lamivudine on transaminases and virologic endpoints. Adapted with permission.[71,72]

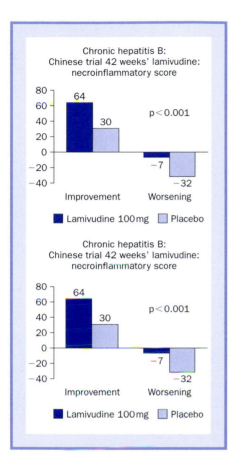

Figure 22.2
Efficacy of lamivudine on necrosis and inflammation in wild-type HBV. Adapted with permission.[71,72]

Biopsy was not performed in the control group, and the results after 48 weeks of treatment were not controlled. However, there was a similar effect to wild-type on necrosis, inflammation and fibrosis worsening (Figure 22.4).

Predictive factors of response

The same factors are associated with a beneficial response to lamivudine as in interferon (Table 22.1). However, there are differences from interferon, as lamivudine seems effective in patients with immunosuppression, patients coinfected with HIV[67,69] or transplanted patients.[75] The biggest difference probably concerns the treatment of patients with decompensated cirrhosis. Lamivudine provides rapid clinical improvement (Figure 22.5).[76,77]

Table 22.1 Factors associated with beneficial response to lamivudine in patients with chronic hepatitis B.

Favorable factors
High serum transaminases activity
Low serum HBV-DNA level
Wild-type (HBeAg-positive) virus?
Absence of immunosuppression?

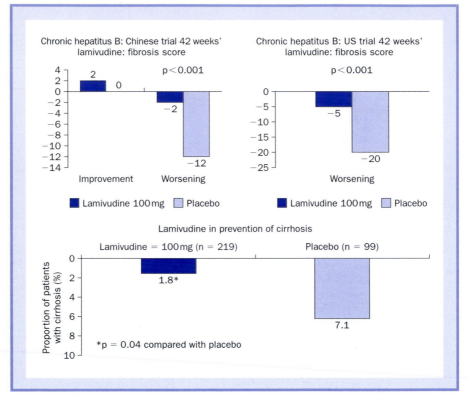

Figure 22.3
Efficacy of lamivudine on fibrosis progression in wild-type HBV. Adapted with permission.[71,72]

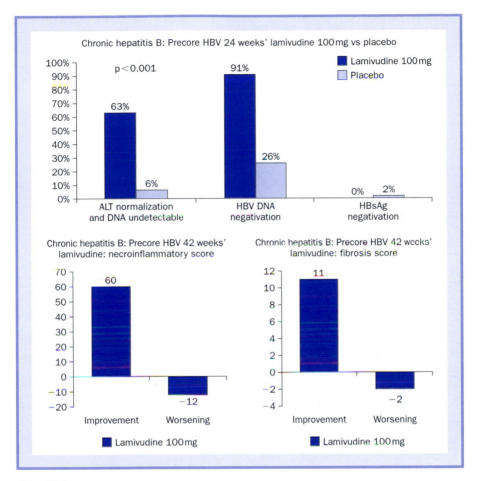

Figure 22.4
Efficacy of lamivudine on transaminases, and virologic and histologic endpoints in precore mutant HBV. Adapted with permission.[73]

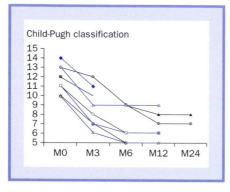

Figure 22.5
Efficacy of lamivudine 100 mg in 13 severely decompensated cirrhotic patients. Adapted with permission.[76]

Incidence of YMDD mutant HBV

The major drawback of lamivudine monotherapy is the emergence of resistant HBV with mutation at the tyrosine-methiomine-aspartate-aspartate (YMDD) motif at the catalytic domain of the viral reverse transcriptase/DNA polymerase.[78–81] The incidence of YMDD mutants rises from 15–30% in the first year to 70% by the fifth year of therapy. Patients with the YMDD mutants tend to have ALT and HBV-DNA levels which are lower than pretreatment levels, probably because the YMDD mutants have less replication competence.[80] A recent study shows that worsening in histology occurs in similar proportions in patients with and without YMDD mutants, but patients

without YMDD mutants are more likely to improve and less likely to deteriorate.[74] However, in some patients, the HBV-DNA levels can become greater than pretreatment levels. This may result in varying degrees of hepatic decompensation.

According to the high relapse rate after 8 months' treatment, at least 48 weeks are recommended. Cessation of treatment in patients with severe liver disease is a major concern, as a flare-up of liver disease is possible, as well as liver failure, due to an uncontrolled replication of wild-type HBV. In patients with severe disease, it is therefore recommended to continue lamivudine and to use adefovir, which is effective on the YMDD mutant.

When to stop lamivudine in patients without severe liver disease

In wild-type HBV, lamivudine can be stopped when there is a HBeAg seroconversion with detectable HBeAb, undetectable HBV DNA by sensitive PCR, and normal transaminases. At least 1 year of treatment is recommended. In precore mutant HBV, lamivudine can be stopped when transaminases are normal and HBV DNA is undetectable. The exact duration of treatment is not clear, but at least 1-year treatment is recommended, as well as at least 1 month with undetectable HBV DNA and normal ALT.

Comparison between lamivudine, interferon and the combination of interferon and lamivudine

23

Several published controlled trials have compared lamivudine 100 mg monotherapy with the combination of interferon and lamivudine.[83-86] The largest study with long-term follow-up included 130 patients in total with an HBeAg seroconversion

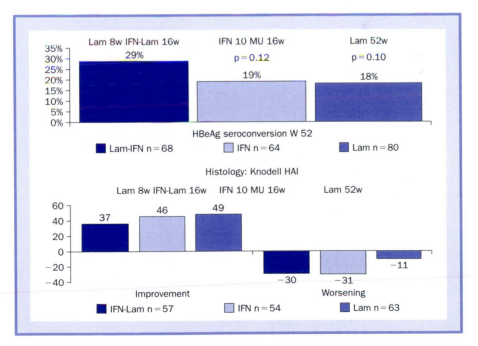

Figure 23.1
Comparison between lamivudine (Lam), interferon (IFN) and interferon and lamivudine combination for HBeAg seroconversion and necrosis and inflammation. Adapted with permission.[84]

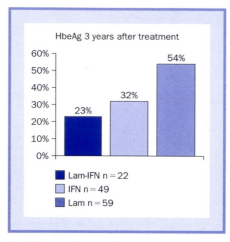

Figure 23.2
Three-year cumulative HBeAg relapse after lamivudine, interferon and lamivudine-interferon combination. Adapted with permission.[86]

(HBeAg negative, antibodies to HBeAg positive) at the end of antiviral therapy. Relapse was defined as confirmed reappearance of HBeAg. The durability of HBeAg seroconversion following lamivudine treatment was significantly lower than that following interferon or interferon-lamivudine combination therapy. The three-year cumulative HBeAg relapse rate was 54% for lamivudine, 32% for interferon, and 23% for combination therapy. The risk of relapse after HBeAg seroconversion was also related to pretreatment levels of serum ALT and HBV DNA, but was independent of Asian race.

One year combination of PEG-IFN alfa-2b and lamivudine gave similar results than PEG-IFN alfa-2b alone.[68]

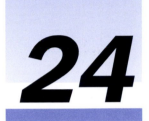

Safety of lamivudine

In general, lamivudine is very well tolerated, with similar occurrence of clinical and biological adverse events in patients receiving lamivudine or placebo (Table 24.1). The main problem is the long-term incidence of mutants. The safety of interferon is discussed in the HCV chapter.

Table 24.1 Serious adverse events in each year. Adapted with permission from GlaxoWellcome.

Therapy	Year of therapy	No. of patients	Patients with severe adverse events		Liver disease related	
			n	%	n	%
Placebo	1st	200	17	8.5	4	2.0
Lam 100 mg	1st	999	42	4.2	7	0.7
Lam 100 mg	2nd	741	24	3.2	15	2.0
Lam 100 mg	3rd	630	26	4.1	12	1.9
Lam 100 mg	4th	208	8	3.8	3	1.4

Efficacy of adefovir

25

Adefovir is the second nucleoside analog to be approved for use in chronic hepatitis B in the United States and in Europe. Adefovir, an acyclic analog of deoxyadenosine monophosphate (dAMP), inhibits the amplification of covalently closed circular DNA (cccDNA) in duck HBV-infected hepatocytes. Adefovir 10 mg daily given for 48 weeks is associated with significantly better histologic improvement, a higher rate of HBeAg seroconversion, a three logarithmic reduction of HBV-DNA levels and a higher chance of normalization of ALT when compared with patients receiving placebo.[87] The same efficacy on HBV DNA and ALT has been observed in another randomized trial of adefovir 10 mg daily given for 48 weeks in patients with HBeAg-negative chronic hepatitis B.[88] In these two trials, there was a very significant histologic improvement with adefovir 10 mg versus placebo (Figure 25.1).

Adefovir dipivoxil is also active against lamivudine-resistant YMDD mutants.[89–94] In these patients with very high baseline viral load, the mean decrease was greater than 2 logs in the first 4 weeks and greater than 3 logs at 24 weeks (Figure 25.2).

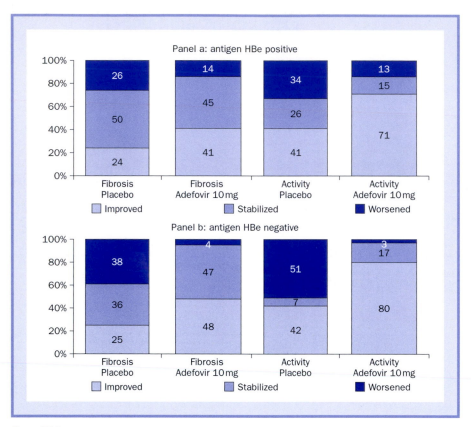

Figure 25.1
*Impact of adefovir 10 mg on fibrosis stage and necroinflammatory activity grade in patients with chronic
hepatitis B: ranked assessment of fibrosis and necroinflammatory scores (percentage of patients). Adapted
with permission.[87,88]*
*Antigen HBe positive (panel a): 168 patients and baseline biopsy treated with adefovir, 161 with placebo
Antigen HBe negative (panel b): 121 patients and baseline biopsy treated with adefovir, 57 with placebo
There was a significant difference (p < 0.001) both for fibrosis and necroinflammatory (activity) scores*

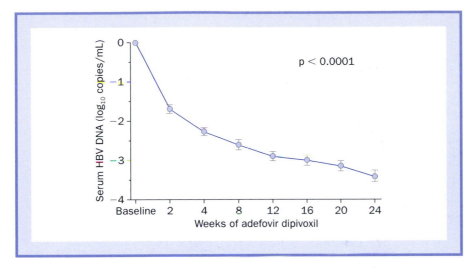

Figure 25.2
Mean changes from baseline in serum HBV DNA measured by PCR during adefovir dipivoxil therapy in HIV/HBV-coinfected patients. Adapted with permission.[93]

Safety of adefovir

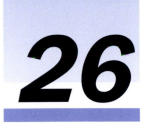

The safety of adefovir is excellent, and is similar to that of lamivudine. When compared to placebo, the nature and frequency of clinical adverse events during the first 48 weeks of the pooled studies were similar between the adefovir dipivoxil 10 mg (0–48 weeks) and placebo groups.[87,88] During the first 48 weeks of treatment in the two double-blind, placebo-controlled studies, 82% of patients in the adefovir dipivoxil 10 mg group experienced at least one adverse event, compared with 85% of patients in the pooled placebo group. In the all adefovir dipivoxil 10 mg group (patients who received at least one dose of adefovir dipivoxil 10 mg at any time in these studies) 69% experienced at least one adverse event.

The most commonly reported adverse events in these groups were headache, pharyngitis, asthenia, abdominal pain and flu syndrome. Among patients in the all adefovir dipivoxil 10 mg group with up to 96 weeks of treatment, the frequency of these events was comparable or lower than the 48-week adefovir dipivoxil 10 mg (0–48 weeks) and placebo groups (Table 26.1).

No renal toxicity has been observed with the 10-mg dose recommended for the treatment of chronic hepatitis B, but renal function must be monitored closely. Mild changes were seen with the 30-mg dose. Adefovir dipivoxil causes proximal renal tubular dysfunction at 6–12 times higher dosages of 60–120 mg used in earlier trials for patients with human immunodeficiency virus (HIV). The changes were mild to moderate and reversible. The renal toxicity is mediated

Table 26.1 Most frequent adverse events (≥3% of patients in the all adefovir dipivoxil 10 mg group): combined studies 437 and 438.

Adverse event	Placebo (0–48) (N = 228)		ADV 10 mg (0–48) (N = 294)		All ADV 10 mg (0–96) (N = 492)	
	n	%	n	%	n	%
Number of patients experiencing adverse events	194	85	242	82	340	69
Headache	47	21	72	24	92	19
Pharyngitis	68	30	67	23	88	18
Asthenia	42	18	58	20	76	15
Abdominal pain	35	15	49	17	75	15
Flu syndrome	44	19	41	14	55	11
Rhinitis	20	9	29	10	43	9
Pain	27	12	29	10	39	8
Diarrhea	15	7	28	10	33	7
Nausea	25	11	22	7	30	6
Back pain	15	7	23	8	29	6
Cough increased	25	11	21	7	28	6
Dyspepsia	16	7	21	7	25	5
Insomnia	14	6	15	5	23	5
Flatulence	12	5	18	6	20	4
Fever	16	7	15	5	20	4
Accidental injury	12	5	12	4	16	3
Myalgia	19	8	10	3	16	3
ALT increased	12	5	9	3	15	3
Rash	18	8	7	2	15	3
Arthralgia	13	6	11	4	14	3
Dizziness	14	6	11	4	14	3
Vomiting	5	2	12	4	14	3

through the human renal organic anion transporter 1.

No adefovir-resistant mutations have been observed up to 135 weeks of treatment. This may be related to the close resemblance of adefovir to its natural substrate and/or the flexible acyclic structure of the adefovir molecule that allows multiple binding modes.[95]

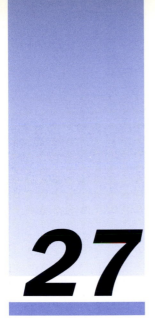

First-line treatment of chronic hepatitis B: Adefovir, lamivudine or interferon?

27

There is no clear consensus on the best treatment except for adefovir or lamivudine in patients with decompensated cirrhosis and in the case of other contraindications to interferon.

In naive patients, there is a choice between adefovir, lamivudine and interferon according to their advantages and disadvantages (Table 27.1).

If the patient prefers oral treatment, one possibility is to start with adefovir. Another possibility is to start with lamivudine and to switch to adefovir if a resistant mutant occurs. If the patient accepts injection, it seems difficult to propose several injections a week and PEG-IFN is probably a better choice.

Table 27.1 Advantages and disadvantages of adefovir, lamivudine and interferon.

Adefovir		Lamivudine		Interferon	
Advantage	*Disadvantage*	*Advantage*	*Disadvantage*	*Advantage*	*Disadvantage*
Oral administration once a day	Long duration of therapy	Oral administration once a day	Long duration of therapy	Short course	Injection
No resistant mutant at 2 years			Resistant mutant (15% per year)	No resistant mutant	
Minimal adverse events	Caution in patients with renal insufficiency	Minimal adverse events			Significant adverse events
Useful in decompensated cirrhosis		Useful in decompensated cirrhosis			Many "problem" patients
Useful in post-transplantation		Useful in post-transplantation			
Fast efficacy on HBV DNA and transaminases	Shorter durability of response?	Fast efficacy on HBV DNA and transaminases	Shorter durability of response?	Longer durability of response?	

New drugs in development

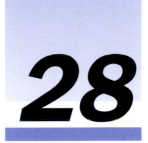

Tenofovir disoproxil fumarate, structurally similar to adefovir and approved for the treatment of HIV, is also effective in suppressing the replication of YMDD mutants.[96–98] Trials must now be performed in patients with the HBV infection alone.

Emtricitabine is similar to lamivudine in structure and potency. Clevudine, a pyrimidine analog, is distinguished by a very slow rebound in HBV-DNA levels after cessation of therapy.[99] Both drugs are ineffective against the YMDD mutants.

Entecavir, a guanosine analog, has a strong inhibitory effect on the priming of HBV polymerase by guanosine triphosphate.[100] No entecavir-resistant mutants have been detected in woodchucks after 3 years of therapy. A phase 2 trial shows that at 6 months, both 0.1 and 0.5 mg daily doses of entecavir are superior to 100 mg of lamivudine in viral suppression.[101] Entecavir, at a higher dose of 1 mg daily, is also effective against YMDD mutants.

Telbuvidine (β-L-2'-deoxythymidine, LdT) is one of three L-nucleosides with specific HBV inhibitory activity.[102] Like lamivudine, which is also a L-nucleoside analog, LdT is almost without side effects. A phase 2 trial shows that, at 6 months, LdT, either alone or in combination with lamivudine, causes significantly better viral suppression than lamivudine monotherapy.[103] LdT 400 and 600 mg daily both cause an unprecedented reduction in median HBV-DNA levels of over 6 $\log_{10}$ at 6 months of therapy.

29

Who needs to be treated and how to explain the goals to the patient

Considering the natural history of hepatitis B, there are four different goals for the treatment:[59,104,105]

1. to prevent the occurrence of cirrhosis and its complications
2. to prevent occurrence of hepatocellular carcinoma, which is possible even in the absence of cirrhosis
3. to reduce the extrahepatic manifestations
4. to prevent the contamination of other people (that is, surgeon or drug user).

Vaccination of relatives is mandatory.

Who need to be treated?

Antiviral therapy is unnecessary in patients with acute hepatitis B. However, studies in severe cases and fulminant hepatitis are necessary.[106] Patients with fulminant hepatitis B should be considered for liver transplantation.

Patients with moderate to severe fibrosis or necroinflammatory activity and active HBV replication should be treated. Patients with decompensated cirrhosis should be treated in specialized liver units.

The utility of a cutoff in HBV replication (that is, HBV-DNA above 10^5 copies/mL) or in transaminases to decide antiviral therapy is controversial.

Patients with extrahepatic manifestations of HBV infection and active replication should be treated. Patients undergoing liver transplantation for hepatitis B should be treated.

Health-care workers with mild chronic hepatitis B should be counseled about the risk and benefit of antiviral therapy. Treatment is recommended for those with HBV replication if they perform procedures that may place patients at risk of HBV infection. There is no general consensus regarding the level below which transmission is unlikely.

Vaccination of contacts is the best way of preventing transmission of HBV in institutionalized persons.

Ten key points for the understanding of the natural history of HBV by patients

1. Almost all the mortality of the disease is related to complications of cirrhosis. Rare cases of primary liver cancer can occur in the absence of cirrhosis.
2. The risk of chronicity varies tremendously with the age of infection. For neonates and children under the age of 1 year who acquire the infection, the risk of chronicity is 90%. For children of 1–5 years of age, the risk is approximately 30%. For children over 5 years old and for adults, the risk decreases to around 2% only.
3. One-third of chronically infected patients will probably never progress to cirrhosis or to cancer.
4. Definition of the healthy carrier (nonactive carrier: normal transaminases, normal histology, no symptoms) is time dependent, and a follow-up is highly recommended.
5. Despite the risk of fibrosis, a patient can be

treated for extrahepatic manifestation or in order to prevent transmission of the virus.
6. Cryoglobulinemia is observed in 10% of cases and is rarely associated with severe symptoms (1% of vasculitis).
7. It is still controversial that viral load and genotype are related to the severity of the disease.
8. Alcohol consumption greater than 4 units a day accelerates the fibrosis progression.
9. Normal transaminases do not exclude the presence of cirrhosis.
10. Relatives can be protected by vaccination.

Ten key points for the understanding of the HBV treatment by patients

1. There are two goals for the treatment of hepatic manifestations: the first goal is to eradicate the virus; if the virus is not eradicated, the second goal is to prevent the progression to cirrhosis, the complications of cirrhosis and the occurrence of primary liver cancer.
2. In wild-type HBV infection (HBeAg positive), the viral response is well defined by undetectable HBV DNA, normal transaminases, undetectable HBeAg and the occurrence of HBeAb (seroconversion HBe).
3. In precore mutant HBV infection (HBeAg negative), the viral response is defined by undetectable HBV DNA and normal transaminases.
4. Seroconversion of HBsAg (undetectable HBsAg and occurrence of HBsAb) occurs rarely after treatment.

5. When a sustained viral response is obtained, there is a dramatic improvement of liver histology, including necroinflammatory features in all patients and fibrosis stage in noncirrhotic patients.

6. When a sustained viral response is obtained in cirrhotic patients, there is a major clinical improvement.

7. Occurrence of lamivudine-resistant mutants is the main concern of this regimen, but a seroconversion can be obtained as well as lower HBV DNA and transaminases in comparison to pretreatment values.

8. Depression and suicide are the most dreadful adverse events of interferon.

9. Adefovir has the same efficacy as lamivudine, without occurrence of resistant mutants after 2 years of therapy.

10. Liver transplantation is no longer contraindicated in patients with HBV cirrhosis.

Management of relapsers and nonresponders

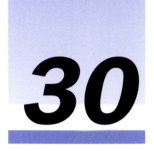

Relapsers and nonresponders to interferon should be treated by adefovir or lamivudine. Relapsers and nonresponders to lamivudine should be treated by adefovir or interferon. Nonresponders to lamivudine are most often patients with a resistant mutant.

Relapsers and nonresponders to adefovir should be treated by lamivudine or interferon. The benefit-risk ratio of the combination of interferon, lamivudine or adefovir is unknown.[107]

Management of patients coinfected by HBV and HIV

31

Among patients infected by HIV, HBV coinfection must be systematically screened, and treatment of HBV must be discussed when fibrosis is observed at liver biopsy. When transaminase activity is increased in a patient infected by HIV with negative HCV PCR, a serum HBV PCR must be performed, as a false-negative HBsAg is possible in immunodepressed patients.

Usually, patients coinfected by HBV and HIV are treated with anti-HIV treatment, including lamivudine. Lamivudine 100 mg monotherapy must not be given to patients infected by HIV, as this dose is ineffective for HIV (300 mg is recommended), and without combined anti-HIV treatment, there is a high risk of a lamivudine-resistant mutant to HIV. Lamivudine-resistant mutant incidence is similar (15% per year) in HIV patients treated with anti-HIV combination in comparison with patients infected by HBV only.[108]

Adefovir 10 mg per day is effective for the treatment of a lamivudine-resistant mutant,[93] as is tenofovir. Tenofovir is effective on both lamivudine-resistant HBV and HIV.[96–98]

If anti-HIV treatment is not indicated, adefovir or interferon can be used as the first-line regimen.

Anti-HIV treatment is often associated with transaminase increase (D4T, DDI, abacavir, nevirapine and protease inhibitor). When the increase is important, another liver biopsy must be discussed and compared to biopsy before treatment. The following factors can be involved: alcohol consumption, illicit IV drug injection, substitution drug toxicity, anti-HIV drug toxicity (mitochondria), coinfection with HCV, HBV or delta virus, liver opportunistic infection, immune restoration and sclerosing cholangitis. The impact of immune reconstitution on liver-fibrosis progression is unknown.

Management of transplanted patients chronically infected by HBV

32

End-stage HBsAg-positive cirrhosis is one of the main indications for orthotopic liver transplantation. Recurrence of HBV infection is the most significant problem, with an 85% rate in the absence of prophylaxis.

During the last 10 years, substantial progress has been made with the passive prophylaxis of hepatitis B immunoglobulin (HBIg),[109] and with the approval of lamivudine and adefovir.[87,88,110,111]

Before transplantation, the best algorithm is to obtain undetectable HBV DNA. The optimal timing of antiviral therapy depends on the patient's condition and expected waiting time for transplantation. Interferon is not recommended because of the poor tolerance in patients with end-stage liver disease. Lamivudine can be started only if transplantation is imminent, that is, less than 6 months. Adefovir is recommended as first-line therapy with monitoring of renal function.

After transplantation, the use of HBIg alone or in combination is controversial. Combination of low-dose HBIg with antiviral therapy, adefovir or lamivudine, seems, so far, to be the best prophylaxis regimen. Breakthrough during lamivudine therapy should be treated with adefovir.

Cost-effectiveness of treatment

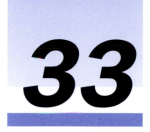

There were reductions in lifetime risk of developing compensated cirrhosis, decompensated cirrhosis and hepatocellular carcinoma of 5%, 11% and 11%, respectively, when lamivudine was available in comparison with interferon.[113] The introduction of lamivudine was expected to reduce and delay the progression of chronic hepatitis B, increasing the life expectancy and quality of life of patients for a small overall increase in health-care costs in comparison with interferon monotherapy (Table 33.1). No cost-effectiveness study of adefovir has been published so far.

Table 33.1 Cost-effectiveness of lamivudine therapy versus interferon. Adapted with permission.[113]

	Lamivudine regimen vs interferon regimen
Life expectancy	
Life expectancy years	3.9 years increase
Quality-adjusted life years	3.2 years increase
Incremental cost	
Per life year	Australian $633 increase
Per quality-adjusted life year	Australian $735 increase

References

1. Blumberg BS, Alter HJ, Visnik S. A "new" antigen in leukemia sera. *JAMA* 1965; **191**: 541–6.

2. Szmuness W, Stevens CE, Hadler SC. Hepatitis B: Evolving epidemiology and implications for control. *Semin Liver Dis* 1991; **11**: 84–92.

3. Maddrey WC. Hepatitis B: An important public health issue. *Clin Lab* 2001; **47**: 51–5.

4. Pawlotsky JM. Molecular diagnosis of viral hepatitis. *Gastroenterology* 2002; **122**: 1554–68.

5. Brechot C, Thiers V, Kremsdorf D, et al. Persistent hepatitis B virus infection in subjects without hepatitis B surface antigen: Clinically significant or purely "occult"? *Hepatology* 2001: **34**: 194–203.

6. Carman WF, Jacyna MR, Hadziyannis S, et al. Mutation preventing formation of hepatitis e antigen in patients with chronic hepatitis B infection. *Lancet* 1989; **2**: 588–91.

7. Bonino F, Brunetto MR, Rizetto M, Will H. Hepatitis B virus unable to secrete e antigen. *Gastroenterology* 1991; **100**: 1138–41.

8. Zarski JP, Marcellin P, Cohard M, et al. Comparison of anti-HBe-positive and HBe-antigen-positive chronic hepatitis B in France. French Multicentre Group. *J Hepatol* 1994; **20**: 636–40.

9. Sanchez-Tapias JM. Natural history of chronic hepatitis B. In M Buti, R Esteban, J Guardia (eds), *Viral Hepatitis*. Barcelona: Accion Medica, 2000, pp. 21–31.

10. Lok ASF. Hepatitis B infection: Pathogenesis and management. *J Hepatol* 2000; **32**: 89–97.

11. Hyams KC. Risks of chronicity following acute hepatitis B virus infection: A review. *Clin Infect Dis* 1995: **20**: 992–1000.

12. Yuen MF, Lai CL. Natural history of chronic hepatitis B virus infection. *J Gastroenterol Hepatol* 2000; **15**(Suppl): E20–4.

13. Reifenberg K, Deutschle T, Wild J, et al. The hepatitis B virus e antigen cannot pass the murine placenta efficiently and does not induce CTL immune tolerance in H-2B mice in utero. *Virology* 1998; **243**: 45–53.

14. Sakuma K, Takahara T, Okuda K, Tsuda F, Mayumi M. Prognosis of hepatitis B virus surface antigen carriers in relation to routine liver function tests: A prospective study. *Gastroenterology* 1982; **83**: 114–17.

15. McMahon BJ, Alberts SR, Wainwright RB, Bulkow L, Lanier AP. Hepatitis B-related sequelae. Prospective study in 1400 hepatitis B surface antigen-positive Alaska native carriers. *Arch Intern Med* 1990; **150**: 1051–4.

16. Bortolotti F, Jara P, Crivellaro C, et al. Outcome of chronic hepatitis B in Caucasian children during a 20-year observation period. *J Hepatol* 1998; **29**: 184–8.

17. Lai ME, Solinas A, Mazzoleni AP, et al. The role of pre-core hepatitis B virus mutants on the long-term outcome of chronic hepatitis B virus hepatitis. A longitudinal study. *J Hepatol* 1994; **20**: 773–81.

18. Poynard T, Mathurin P, Lai CL, et al. A comparison of fibrosis progression in chronic liver diseases. *J Hepatol* 2003; **38**: 257–65.

19. Hoofnagle JH, Shafritz DA, Popper H. Chronic type B hepatitis and the "healthy" HBsAg carrier state. *Hepatology* 1987; **7**: 758–63.

20. Martinot-Peignoux M, Boyer N, Colombat M, et al. Serum hepatitis B virus DNA levels and liver histology in inactive HBsAg carriers. *J Hepatol* 2002; **36**: 543–6.

21. Chu CJ, Hussain M, Lok ASF. Quantitative serum HBV DNA levels during different stages of chronic hepatitis B infection. *Hepatology* 2002; **36**: 1408–15.

22. Yuen MF, Sablon E, Hui CK, et al. Prognostic factors in severe exacerbation of chronic hepatitis B. *Clin Infect Dis* 2003 (in press).

23. Yuen MF, Sablon E, Yuan HJ, et al.

Relationship between the development of precore and core promoter mutations and hepatitis B e antigen seroconversion in patients with chronic hepatitis B virus. *J Infect Dis* 2002; **186**: 1335–8.

24. Chan HL, Leung NW, Hussain M, Wong ML, Lok ASK. Hepatitis B e antigen-negative chronic hepatitis B in Hong Kong. *Hepatology* 2000; **31**: 763–8.

25. Sanchez-Tapias JM, Costa J, Mas A, Bruguera M, Rodes M. Influence of hepatitis B virus genotype on the long-term outcome of chronic hepatitis B in Western patients. *Gastroenterology* 2002; **123**: 1848–56.

26. Chu CJ, Hussain M, Lok ASF. Hepatitis B virus genotype B is associated with earlier HBeAg seroconversion compared with hepatitis B virus genotype C. *Gastroenterology* 2002; **122**: 1756–62.

27. Kao JH, Wu NH, Chen PJ, Lai MY, Chen DS. Hepatitis B genotypes and the response to interferon therapy. *J Hepatol* 2000; **33**: 998–1002.

28. Wai CY, Chu CJ, Hussain M, Lok AS. HBV genotype B is associated with a higher response rate to interferon therapy than genotype C. *Hepatology* 2002; **36**: 1425–30.

29. Yuen MF, Sablon E, Yuan HJ, et al. The significance of hepatitis B genotype in acute exacerbation, HBeAg seroconversion, cirrhosis-related complications and hepatocellular carcinoma. *Hepatology* 2003 (in press).

30. Orito E, Ichida T, Sakugawa H, et al. Geographic distribution of hepatitis B (HBV) genotype in patients with chronic HBV infection in Japan. *Hepatology* 2001; **34**: 590–4.

31. Sumi H, Yokosuka O, Seki N, et al. Influence of hepatitis B virus genotypes on the progression of chronic type B liver disease. *Hepatology* 2003; **37**: 19–26.

32. Villeneuve JP, Desrochers M, Infante-Rivard C, et al. A long-term follow-up study of asymptomatic hepatitis B surface antigen-positive carriers in Montreal. *Gastroenterology* 1994; **106**: 1000–5.

33. de Franchis R, Meucci G, Vecchi M, et al.

The natural history of asymptomatic hepatitis B surface antigen carriers. *Ann Intern Med* 1993; **118**: 191–4.

34. Tsubota A, Kumada H, Takaki K, et al. Deletions in the hepatitis B virus core gene may influence the clinical outcome in hepatitis B e antigen-positive asymptomatic healthy carriers. *J Med Virol* 1998; **56**: 287–93.

35. Tainturier-Sayegh MH, Thibault V, Ratziu V, et al. Is it possible to reduce liver biopsy indication in HBsAg-positive patients with undetectable HBV-DNA? *Hepatology* 2000; **32**: 452A.

36. Huo TI, Wu JC, Lee PC, et al. Sero-clearance of hepatitis B surface antigen in chronic carriers does not necessarily imply a good prognosis. *Hepatology* 1998; **28**: 231–6.

37. Beasley RP, Hwang LY, Lin CC, Chien CS. Hepatocellular carcinoma and hepatitis B virus. A prospective study of 22,707 men in Taiwan. *Lancet* 1981; **2**: 1129–33.

38. Okuda K. Early recognition of hepatocellular carcinoma. *Hepatology* 1986: **6**: 729–38.

39. Bosch X. Global epidemiology of hepatocellular carcinoma. In K Okuda, E Tabor (eds), *Liver Cancer*. New York: Churchill Livingstone, 1997: pp. 13–28.

40. Brechot C, Hadchouel M, Scotto J, et al. State of hepatitis B virus DNA in hepatocytes of patients with HBsAg positive and HBsAg negative liver diseases. *Proc Natl Acad Sci USA* 1981; **78**: 3906–10.

41. Popper H, Shih JW, Gerin JL, et al. Woodchuck hepatitis and hepatocellular carcinoma: Correlation of histological and virological observations. *Hepatology* 1981: **1**: 91–98.

42. El-Serag HB, Mason A. Rising incidence of hepatocellular carcinoma in the United States. *N Engl J Med* 1999; **34**: 745–50.

43. Chang MH, Chen CJ, Lai MS, et al. Universal hepatitis B vaccination in Taiwan and the incidence of hepatocellular carcinoma in children. *N Engl J Med* 1997; **336**: 1855–9.

44. Chen PJ, Chen DS. Hepatitis B virus infection and hepatocellular carcinoma:

Molecular genetics and clinical perspectives. *Semin Liver Dis* 1999; **19**: 253–62.

45. Cacciola I, Pollicino T, Squadrito G, et al. Occult hepatitis B virus infection in patients with chronic hepatitis C liver disease. *N Engl J Med* 1999; **341**: 22–6.

46. Yamamoto K, Horikita M, Tsuda F, et al. Naturally occurring escape mutants of hepatitis B virus with various mutations in the S gene in carriers seropositive for antibody to hepatitis B surface antigen. *J Virol* 1994; **68**: 2671–6.

47. Rehermann B, Ferrari C, Pasquinelli C, Chisari FV. The hepatitis B virus persists for decades after patients' recovery from acute viral hepatitis despite active maintenance of a cytotoxic T-lymphocyte response. *Nat Med* 1996; **2**: 1104–8.

48. Trepo C, Thivolet J. Antigène Australia antigen, virus de l'hépatite et periarterite noueuse. *Presse Med* 1970; **78**: 1575.

49. Willson RA. Extrahepatic manifestations of chronic viral hepatitis. In RA Willson (ed.) *Viral Hepatitis, Diagnostic, Treatment, Prevention*. New York: Marcel Dekker, 1997, pp. 331–69.

50. Pyrsopoulos NT, Reddy KR. Extrahepatic manifestations of chronic viral hepatitis. *Curr Gastroenterol Rep* 2001; **3**: 71–8.

51. Lhote F, Cohen P, Guillevin L. Polyarteritis nodosa, microscopic polyangiitis and Churg-Strauss syndrome. *Lupus* 1998; **7**: 238–58.

52. Guillevin L, Lhote F, Cohen P, et al. Polyarteritis nodosa related to hepatitis B virus. A prospective study with long-term observation of 41 patients. *Medicine (Baltimore)* 1995; **74**: 238–53.

53. Zurn A, Schmied E, Saurat JH. Cutaneous manifestations of infection due to hepatitis B virus. *Schweiz Rundsch Med Prax* 1990; **79**: 1254–7.

54. Johnson RJ, Gouser WG. Hepatitis B infection and renal disease: Clinical, immunopathogenic and therapeutic considerations. *Kidney Int* 1990; **37**: 663–76.

55. Lunel F, Musset L, Cacoub P, et al. Cryoglobulinemia in chronic liver diseases:

Role of hepatitis C virus and liver damage. *Gastroenterology* 1994; **106**: 1291–300.

56. Foster GR, Goldin RD, Thomas HC. Chronic hepatitis C virus infection causes a significant reduction in quality of life in the absence of cirrhosis. *Hepatology* 1998; **27**: 209–12.

57. Owens DK, Cardinalli AB, Nease RF. Physicians' assessments of the utility of health states associated with human immunodeficiency virus (HIV) and hepatitis B virus (HBV) infection. *Qual Life Res* 1997; **6**: 77–86.

58. Hoofnagle JH, di Bisceglie AM. The treatment of chronic viral hepatitis. *N Engl J Med* 1997; **336**: 347–56.

59. Lai CL, Yuen MF, Locarnini S. Treatment of chronic hepatitis B infection. In CL Lai, S Locarnini (eds), *A Guide to Hepatitis B Virus.* International Medical Press, 2003 (in press).

60. Myers RP, Tainturier MH, Ratziu V, et al. Prediction of liver histological lesions with biochemical markers in patients with chronic hepatitis B. *J Hepatol* 2003; **39**: 222–30.

61. Wong DK, Cheung AM, O'Rourke K, et al. Effect of alpha-interferon treatment in patients with hepatitis B e antigen-positive chronic hepatitis B. A meta-analysis. *Ann Intern Med* 1993; **119**: 312–23.

62. Brook MG, Petrovic L, McDonald JA, Scheuer PJ, Thomas HC. Histological improvement after anti-viral treatment for chronic hepatitis B virus infection. *J Hepatol* 1989; **8**: 218–25.

63. Niederau C, Heintges T, Lange S, et al. Long-term follow-up of HBeAg-positive patients treated with interferon alfa for chronic hepatitis B. *N Engl J Med* 1996; **334**: 1422–7.

64. Lin SM, Sheen IS, Chien RN, Chu CM, Liaw YF. Long-term beneficial effect of interferon therapy in patients with chronic hepatitis B virus infection. *Hepatology* 1999; **29**: 971–5.

65. Yuen MF, Hui CK, Cheng CC, et al. Long-term follow-up of interferon-alpha treatment in Chinese patients with chronic hepatitis B infection: The effect on HBeAg seroconversion and the development of cirrhosis-related complications. *Hepatology* 2001; **34**: 785–91.

66. Perrillo R, Tamburro C, Regenstein F, et al. Low-dose, titratable interferon alpha in decompensated liver disease caused by chronic infection with hepatitis B virus. *Gastroenterology* 1995; **109**: 908–16.

67. Cooksley WGE, Piravisuth T, Wang YJ, et al. Peginterferon alfa-2A: Efficacy and safety results from phase II, randomised, actively controlled, multicenter study in the treatment of HBeAg positive chronic hepatitis B [Abstract]. *Hepatology* 2001; **34**: 349A.

68. Janssen HLA, Senturk H, Zeuzem S, et al. Peginterferon therapy compared with peginterferon alfa-2b for chronic HBeAg-positive Hepatitis B. A randomized controlled trial in 307 patients. *Hepatology* 2003; **38**: 1323.

69. Benhamou Y, Dohin E, Lunel-Fabiani F, et al. Efficacy of lamivudine on replication of hepatitis B virus in HIV-infected patients [Letter]. *Lancet* 1995; **345**: 396–7.

70. Dienstag JL, Perrillo RP, Schiff ER, et al. A preliminary trial of lamivudine for chronic hepatitis B infection. *N Engl J Med* 1995; **333**: 1657–61.

71. Lai CL, Chien RN, Leung NWY, et al. A one year trial of lamivudine for chronic hepatitis B. *N Engl J Med* 1998; **339**: 61–8.

72. Dienstag JL, Schiff ER, Wright T, et al. Lamivudine as initial treatment for chronic hepatitis B in the United States. *N Engl J Med* 1999; **341**: 1256–63.

73. Tassopoulos NC, Volpes R, Pastore G, et al. Efficacy of lamivudine in patients with hepatitis B e antigen-negative/hepatitis B virus DNA-positive (precore mutant) chronic hepatitis B. *Hepatology* 1999; **29**: 889–96.

74. Dienstag JL, Goldin RD, Heathcote EJ, et al. Histological outcome during long-term lamivudine therapy. *Gastroenterology* 2003; **124**: 105–17.

75. Perrillo R. Multicenter study of lamivudine therapy for hepatitis B after liver transplantation. Lamivudine Transplant Group. *Hepatology* 1999; **29**: 1581–6.

76. Yao FY, Bass NM. Lamivudine treatment in patients with severely decompensated cirrhosis

due to replicating hepatitis B infection. *J Hepatol* 2000; **33**: 301–7.

77. Yao FY, Terrault NA, Freise C, Maslow L, Bass NM. Lamivudine treatment is beneficial in patients with severely decompensated cirrhosis and actively replicating hepatitis B infection awaiting liver transplantation: A comparative study using a matched, untreated cohort. *Hepatology* 2001; **34**: 411–16.

78. Liaw YF, Lai CL, Leung NWY, et al. Effects of extended lamivudine therapy in Asian patients with chronic hepatitis B. *Gastroenterology* 2000; **119**: 172–80.

79. Chayama K, Suzuki Y, Kobayashi M, et al. Emergence and takeover of YMDD motif mutant hepatitis B virus during long-term lamivudine therapy and re-takeover by wild type after cessation of therapy. *Hepatology* 1998; **27**: 1711–16.

80. Allen MI, Deslauriers M, Andrews CW, et al. Identification and characterization of mutations in hepatitis B virus resistant to lamivudine. Lamivudine Clinical Investigation Group. *Hepatology* 1998; **27**: 1670–7.

81. Lai CL, Dienstag JL, Schiff E, et al. Prevalence and clinical correlates of YMDD variants during lamivudine therapy of patients with chronic hepatitis B. *Clin Infect Dis* 2003.

82. Dienstag JL, Goldin RD, Heathcote EJ, et al. Histological outcome during long-term lamivudine therapy. *Gastroenterology* 2003; **124**; 105–17.

83. Schalm SW, Heathcote J, Cianciara J, et al., and International Lamivudine Study Group. Lamivudine and alpha interferon combination treatment of patients with chronic hepatitis B infection: A randomised trial. *Gut* 2000; **46**: 562–8.

84. Santantonio T, Niro GA, Sinisi E, et al. Lamivudine/interferon combination therapy in anti-HBe positive chronic hepatitis B patients: A controlled pilot study. *J Hepatol* 2002; **36**: 799–804.

85. Barbaro G, Zechini F, Pellicelli AM, et al. Long-term efficacy of interferon alpha-2b and lamivudine in combination compared to lamivudine monotherapy in patients with chronic hepatitis B. An Italian multicenter, randomized trial. *J Hepatol* 2001; **35**: 406–11.

86. van Nunen AB, Hansen BE, Suh DJ, et al. Durability of HBeAg seroconversion following antiviral therapy for chronic hepatitis B: Relation to type of therapy and pretreatment serum hepatitis B virus DNA and alanine aminotransferase. *Gut* 2003; **52**: 420–4.

87. Marcellin P, Chang TT, Lim SG, et al., and the Adefovir Dipivoxil 437 Study Group. Adefovir dipivoxil for the treatment of HBeAg-positive chronic hepatitis B. *N Engl J Med* 2003; **348**: 808–16.

88. Hadziyannis SJ, Tassopoulos NC, Heathcote J, et al., and the Adefovir Dipivoxil 438 Study Group. Adefovir dipivoxil for the treatment of patients with hepatitis B e antigen-negative chronic hepatitis B. *N Engl J Med* 2003; **348**: 800–7.

89. Das K, Xiong X, Yang H, et al. Molecular modeling and biochemical characterization reveal the mechanism of hepatitis B virus polymerase resistance to lamivudine (3TC) and emtricitabine (FTC). *J Virol* 2001; **75**: 4771–9.

90. Ying C, De Clercq E, Nicholson W, Furman P, Neyts J. Inhibition of the replication of the DNA polymerase M550V mutation variant of human hepatitis B virus by adefovir, tenofovir, L-FMAU, DAPD, penciclovir and lobucavir. *J Viral Hepat* 2000; **7**: 161–5.

91. Xiong K, Flores C, Yang H, Toole JJ, Gibbs CS. Mutations in hepatitis B DNA polymerase associated with resistance to lamivudine do not confer resistance to adefovir *in vitro*. *Hepatology* 1998; **28**: 1669–73.

92. Perrillo R, Schiff E, Yoshida E, et al. Adefovir dipivoxil for the treatment of lamivudine-resistant hepatitis B mutants. *Hepatology* 2000; **32**: 129–34.

93. Benhamou Y, Bochet M, Thibault V, et al. Safety and efficacy of adefovir dipivoxil in patients co-infected with HIV-1 and lamivudine-resistant hepatitis B virus: An open-label pilot study. *Lancet* 2001; **358**: 718–23.

94. Peters MG, Singer G, Howard T, et al. Fulminant hepatic failure resulting from lamivudine-resistant B virus in a renal transplant recipient: Durable response after orthotopic liver transplantation on adefovir dipivoxil and hepatitis B immune globulin. *Transplantation* 1999; **68**: 1912–14.

95. Ono SK, Kato N, Shiratori Y, et al. The polymerase L528M mutation cooperates with nucleotide binding-site mutations, increasing hepatitis B virus replication and drug resistance. *J Clin Invest* 2001; **107**: 449–55.

96. Ying C, De Clerq E, Nicholson W, Furman P, Neyts J. Inhibition of the replication of the DNA polymerase M550V mutation variant of human hepatitis B virus by adefovir, tenofovir, L-FMAU, DAPD, penciclovir and lobucavir. *J Viral Hepat* 2000; 7: 161–5.

97. van Bommel F, Wunsche T, Schurmann D, Berg T. Tenofovir treatment in patients with lamivudine-resistant hepatitis B mutants strongly affects viral replication. *Hepatology* 2002; **36**: 507–8.

98. Benhamou Y, Tubiana R, Thibault V. Tenofovir disoproxil fumarate in patients with HIV and lamivudine-resistant hepatitis B virus [Letter]. *N Engl J Med* 2003; **348**: 177–8.

99. Chu CK, Boudinot FD, Peek SF, et al. Preclinical investigation of L-FMAU as an anti-hepatitis B virus agent. *Antivir Ther* 1998 (Suppl 3): 113–21.

100. Colonno RJ, Genovesi EV, Medina I, et al. Long-term entecavir treatment results in sustained antiviral efficacy and prolonged life span in the woodchuck model of chronic hepatitis infection. *J Infect Dis* 2001; **184**: 1236–45.

101. Lai CL, Rosmawati M, Lao J, et al. Entecavir is superior to lamivudine in reducing hepatitis B virus DNA in patients with chronic hepatitis B infection. *Gastroenterology* 2002; **123**: 1831–8.

102. Bryant ML, Bridges EG, Placidi L, et al. Antiviral L-nucleosides specific for hepatitis B virus infection. *Antimicrob Agents Chemother* 2001; **45**: 229–35.

103. Lai CL, Leung N, Teo EK, et al. International multicenter trial of LdT (telbivudine) alone and in combination with lamivudine, for chronic hepatitis B: An interim analysis. *Hepatology* 2002; **36**: 301A.

104. Valla C. The EASL jury. EASL International Consensus Conference on Hepatitis B. *J Hepatol* 2003: **39**: 533–40.

105. Conjeevaram HS, Lok ASF. Management of chronic hepatitis B. *J Hepatol* 2003; **38**: S90–103.

106. Santantonio T, Mazzola M, Pastore G. Lamivudine is safe and effective in fulminant hepatitis B. *J Hepatol* 1999; **30**: 551.

107. Schalm S, De Man R, Janssen H. Combination and newer therapies for chronic hepatitis B. *J Gastroenterol Hepatol* 2002; 17(Suppl 3): S338–41.

108. Benhamou Y, Katlama C, Lunel F, et al. Effects of lamivudine on replication of hepatitis B virus in HIV-infected men. *Ann Intern Med* 1996; **125**: 705–12.

109. Shouval D, Samuel D. Hepatitis B immune globulin to prevent hepatitis B virus graft reinfection following liver transplantation: A concise review. *Hepatology* 2000; **32**: 1189–95.

110. Colquhoun SD, Belle SH, Samuel D, Pruett TL, Teperman LW. Transplantation in the hepatitis B patient and current therapies to prevent recurrence. *Semin Liver Dis* 2000; **20**(Suppl 1): 7–12.

111. Perrillo RP, Wright T, Rakela J, et al. A multicenter United States–Canadian trial to assess lamivudine monotherapy before and after liver transplantation for chronic hepatitis B. *Hepatology* 2001; **33**: 424–32.

112. Han SH, Ofman J, Holt C, et al. An efficacy and cost-effectiveness analysis of combination hepatitis B immune globulin and lamivudine to prevent recurrent hepatitis B after orthotopic liver transplantation compared with hepatitis B immune globulin monotherapy. *Liver Transpl* 2000; **6**: 741–8.

113. Crowley SJ, Tognarini D, Desmond PV, Lees M. Cost-effectiveness analysis of lamivudine for the treatment of chronic hepatitis B. *Pharmacoeconomics* 2000; **17**: 409–27.

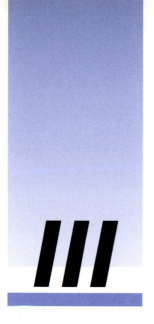

Biochemical markers:
an alternative to liver biopsies

Needle biopsy of the liver: Value and limitations

34

From 1900 to 2002, the liver biopsy was considered the "gold standard" for assessing the stage and the grade of chronic liver diseases. The consensus conference statements recommended liver biopsy in the management of almost all patients with chronic hepatitis B (Table 34.2)[1–10] and C (Table 34.1). The regulatory approvals in Europe, but not in the USA, also asked for liver biopsy in the indications of hepatitis B and C treatments (Table 34.3).

In 2002, for the first time, the consensus conferences in France and the USA started to mention the possibility of treating patients with chronic hepatitis C without liver biopsy.[7,8] These two last conferences also underlined the necessity of developing reliable noninvasive tests that might be an alternative to liver biopsy in both hepatitis B[10] (Table 34.2) and C[7,8] (Table 34.1).

If hepatologists consider liver biopsy to be an essential procedure in making rational decisions,[11–13] patients and general practitioners may consider it an invasive procedure.[14,15] Therefore, there is a risk of reduction of treatment indication in diseases such as chronic hepatitis B or C, despite very effective drugs.

This chapter aims to review the advantages and limits of histologic and biochemical markers of liver features in chronic viral hepatitis B and C.

Table 34.1 Differences between consensus statements on liver biopsy and biochemical markers in chronic hepatitis C.

Biopsy statements	NIH 1997	EASL 1999	France 2002	NIH 2002
General statement	Gold standard Assessment of grade and stage Excludes other diseases	Appropriate and important Assessment of grade and stage	Crucial in most cases	Unique source information Useful part of informed consent project
Recommended before treatment	Indicated when histologic findings will assist decision making regarding patient management	All patients	Not all	Not all Assessment of grade and stage Exclude other diseases
Not recommended before treatment	When histologic findings will not assist decision making regarding patient management	None	Not necessary if the decision to treat has already been taken and does not depend on histologic results Genotypes 2 or 3 Women planning to become pregnant Symptomatic cryoglobulinemia HCV-HIV when antiretroviral treatment can be postponed Clinical, biological and sonographic signs of cirrhosis	Not always necessary in patients of genotypes 2 or 3
Indication of treatment	Either portal or bridging fibrosis and at least moderate degrees of inflammation and necrosis	Moderate/severe necro-inflammation and/or fibrosis	Bridging fibrosis	Either portal or bridging fibrosis, and at least moderate degrees of inflammation and necrosis
Patients with normal transaminases	Liver biopsies can show chronic hepatitis in many of these patients	Not routine recommended, although 20% of them have significant liver disease	Not recommended	Experts differ on whether to biopsy patients with normal ALT levels
Patients with cirrhosis	No statement	No statement	Not recommended	No statement
Follow-up in nontreated patients	Assess disease progression Every 3 to 5 years	Necessary to assess progression of fibrosis Repeat liver biopsy at interval of 4–5 years is recommended	Not recommended before 5 years unless transaminase levels increase or cofactor	Valuable standard for subsequent comparisons The appropriate interval for subsequent histologic evaluations is yet to be determined
Follow-up in treated patients	Not necessary	Repeat biopsy not necessary	Not required in sustained responder	No statement
Safety	Some morbidity	No statement	Side effects need to be more clearly described	No statement
Cost	Expensive	No statement	No statement	No statement
Surrogate markers of fibrosis	No statement	Theme of the future	Serum markers of fibrosis might become an alternative to liver biopsy if they are validated in ongoing studies	Specific serum markers of fibrosis or inflammation not currently available or well validated Research strongly encouraged

Table 34.2 Differences between consensus statements on liver biopsy and biochemical markers in chronic hepatitis B

Biopsy statements	2000 workshop	EASL 2002
General statement	Warranted to assess the grade and stage	Integral part of diagnosis and management Confirming diagnosis, identifying other causes Assessment of grade and stage
Recommended before treatment	Patients with elevated transaminases	All patients Liver biopsy is most helpful in HBV-HIV-coinfected patients
Not recommended before treatment	No biopsy and no treatment for patients with normal transaminases	No statement
Indication of treatment	Moderate activity and fibrosis	Moderate to severe chronic hepatitis; moderate to severe necroinflammation; and fibrosis Mild chronic hepatitis (absence or minimal inflammation) should be monitored. Although the stage of fibrosis is probably related to cumulative activity over time, it should not be considered in evaluating the grade of ongoing activity
Patients with normal transaminases	Liver biopsy is not necessary unless there is other evidence for significant underlying or ongoing liver disease	Cirrhosis may be present in patients with normal transaminases and low or undetectable HBV DNA
Patients with cirrhosis	No statement	Cirrhosis may be present in patients with normal transaminases and low or undetectable HBV DNA
Follow-up in nontreated patients	Repeat liver biopsy not needed unless therapy is considered	May be performed to confirm progression to moderate or severe hepatitis. The required frequency depends on the overall severity of the disease
Follow-up in treated patients	Repeat liver biopsy not needed	Criteria used in trials may not be clinically relevant because of sampling error and interobserver variability Not clear whether repeated biopsy has any benefit. Decision should be made on a case-by-case basis, depending on the likelihood that the findings will affect management
Safety	No statement	Patients should be advised of the benefits, limitations, and the risks and discomfort of liver biopsy
Cost	No statement	No statement
Surrogate markers of fibrosis	No statement	We need reliable noninvasive tests as alternative to liver biopsy

Historical experience over 120 years

The initiation of liver biopsy, in 1883, is attributed in the literature to P. Ehrlich, quoted by von Frerichs,[1] the first series of biopsies being published in 1907.[4] The first evaluation had been published in 1935 by P. Huard,[3] but a milestone in the professionalization of this technique was the publication by G. Menghini of his famous needle procedure in 1958[4] (Table 34.4).

Fibrosis and necroinflammatory activity

Current understanding of chronic hepatitis infection has been advanced, first, by the separation of fibrosis staging and necroinflammatory histologic activity grading[16–20] (Table 34.5), and, second, by the concept of liver fibrosis progression.[21–24]

Fibrosis is the deleterious but variable consequence of chronic inflammation. It is characterized by the deposition of extracellular matrix components, leading to the distortion of the hepatic architecture with impairment of microcirculation and cell functions in the liver. HCV is usually lethal only when it leads to cirrhosis, the last stage of liver fibrosis. Therefore, an estimation of fibrosis progression represents an important surrogate endpoint for evaluation of the vulnerability of an individual patient and for assessment of the impact of treatment on natural history.

One advantage of liver biopsy is that it describes not only fibrosis and necrotico-inflammatory histologic activity but also possible associated disorders such as steatosis, iron overload or nonalcoholic steatohepatitis.

Limitations

No scoring system has so far integrated a definition of normal liver into its own definitions. It is only very recently that the standards of the normal liver have been established.[25,26]

Sampling error

Clinicians who work closely with pathologists soon recognize the pitfalls of sampling errors and the need to obtain adequate biopsy specimens. As stated by Klatskin and Conn, "We are convinced that lack of experience is a much less serious handicap for pathologists than having to interpret sections that are too small or fragmented or poorly prepared".[27]

Experienced pathologists have stated that the reliable interpretation requires at least an unfragmented core of liver 1–2 cm in length. A recent study has established that 2.5 cm in length is necessary[28] for correct classification in fibrosis staging or activity grading.

In the last 33 years, several studies have assessed the sampling variability[28–38] (Table 34.6). When laparoscopic biopsy from the right lobe was compared to biopsy of the left lobe in 80 alcoholic patients, the overall concordance rate was 70%, including 73% for the staging of fibrosis.[30] When three percutaneous biopsies were performed, in 75 patients with different liver diseases, by a single entry site, the overall concordance rate was only 51%.[31]

In 124 patients with chronic hepatitis C, a recent study using laparoscopy observed discordance of at least one grade between the right and left lobes in 30 cases (24.2%), and a discordance of at least one stage in 41 cases

Table 34.3 Differences between indications approved for recent treatments in chronic viral hepatitis in Europe or the USA.

	HCV: PEG-IFN ribavirin		HBV: adefovir	
	Europe	*USA*	*Europe*	*USA*
Clinic	Chronic hepatitis C including patients with compensated cirrhosis	Chronic hepatitis C patients who have compensated liver disease	Chronic hepatitis B Compensated Or decompensated liver disease	Chronic hepatitis B
Virus	Positive for HCV RNA or anti-HCV		With evidence of active viral replication	With evidence of active viral replication
Histology	And histologically proven chronic hepatitis C		And histological evidence of active liver inflammation and fibrosis	And histologically active disease
Biochemistry	Or elevated transaminases since 2003		And persistent elevation in serum aminotransferases	*Or* persistent elevation in serum aminotransferases

Table 34.4 Milestones in liver biopsy for chronic viral hepatitis.

1883	First liver biopsy
1935	First series of liver biopsies
1958	One-second needle biopsy
1981	Knodell staging and grading
1994	METAVIR staging and grading

(33.1%).[34] In 18 patients (14.5%), an interpretation of cirrhosis was given for one lobe, whereas stage 3 fibrosis was given for the other. A difference of two stages or two grades was found in three (2.4%) and two (1.6%) patients, respectively. All the biopsy samples were greater than 15 mm with five or more portal zones and one fragment.

False-positive results in fibrosis staging with percutaneous liver biopsy

Surgical wedge biopsies are at risk of false-positive finding of extensive fibrosis due to the subcapsular normal fibrosis as well as artifact necrosis and neutrophils.[35] If laparoscopic appearance is considered the gold standard for cirrhosis diagnosis, the specificity of biopsy varied from 50%[36] to 99%.[38]

False-negative results in fibrosis staging with percutaneous liver biopsy

If laparoscopic appearance is considered the gold standard for cirrhosis diagnosis, the sensitivity of a right lobe biopsy was 77% (37 out of 48 patients) and 91% for the left lobe biopsy (44 out of 48) in a study in alcoholic liver disease.[30] with laparoscopy as the gold standard, the sensitivity of liver biopsy was 68% in 434 patients with mixed liver diseases.[37] If autopsy histology is considered the gold standard for cirrhosis diagnosis, the sensitivity of three intercostal biopsies was 75% (15 out of 20 patients).[31]

Discordance between pathologists

In chronic liver disease, several studies have evaluated the intra- and interobserver (pathologist) concordance.[18,29,34,39–41] For viral chronic liver disease, the interobserver concordance was better for fibrosis stages (substantial kappa statistic around 0.70–0.80) than for activity grades (moderate kappa statistic around 0.40–0.50). The more detailed Ishak fibrosis scoring system seems less reproducible than the scoring system using five stages only.[39] The intraobserver

Table 34.5 Staging hepatic fibrosis: most often used scoring systems.

Fibrosis	Knodell et al.	METAVIR Bedossa et al.	Ishak et al.
None	0	0	0
Portal fibrosis (some)	1	1	1
Portal fibrosis (most)	1	1	2
Bridging fibrosis (few)	3	2	3
Bridging fibrosis (many)	3	3	4
Incomplete cirrhosis	4	4	4
Cirrhosis	4	4	6

Table 34.6 Sampling error of percutaneous liver biopsies.

First author	Patients	First sample	Other samples	Concordance rate (one stage)
Labayle et al.	80 patients with alcoholic liver disease	Right lobe	Left lobe	Six stages score 44% Cirrhosis 77%
Maharaj et al.	75 patients with mixed liver diseases	One sample	Two other samples single entry site	Cirrhosis 50%
Abdi et al.	118 patients died with mixed liver diseases	One sample	Two other samples	Cirrhosis 75%
Regev et al.	124 patients with chronic hepatitis C	Right lobe	Left lobe	Fibrosis stage 67% Cirrhosis 85% Activity grade 76%
Bedossa et al.	17 patients with chronic hepatitis C 10 659 virtual biopsies	Virtual 15 mm Virtual 25 mm	Virtual 15 mm Virtual 25 mm	Fibrosis stage 65% Fibrosis stage 75%

Table 34.7 Interobserver concordance in liver biopsy staging and grading for chronic hepatitis C.

First author	Patients	METAVIR fibrosis stage	Cirrhosis	Knodell fibrosis stage	Ishak fibrosis stage	METAVIR activity grade	Knodell activity grade
Bedossa et al.	30 patients	0.80	0.91	0.78		0.56	0.48
Westin et al.	95 patients			0.49	0.26–0.47		0.11–0.41
Gronbaek et al.	46 biopsies from 20 patients	0.69			0.51	0.72	0.40

concordance was also found to be greater for fibrosis staging than for activity grading in one study,[18] but not in a recent one.[34]

The interobserver agreement obtained with 100 thin-needle biopsies was significantly lower than the agreement obtained with large-needle biopsies as control. Kappa values for staging were fair (kappa = 0.351) and ranged from slight to fair in agreement (0.003–0.419) for the necroinflammation features.[42]

Adverse events of percutaneous liver biopsy

A summary of the published studies (with more than 200 patients) assessing severe adverse events and mortality rates is given in Table 34.8.[15,43–51] The observed severe adverse events rate was 3/1000. There was a significant heterogeneity among the observed mortality rates, mean 0.3/1000, with a range from 0 to 3.3/1000. The risk factors identified were age and cirrhosis.

Cost of liver biopsy

The cost of liver biopsy is estimated at US$1032 without complications and at US$2745 with complications.[52]

Discordance between clinicians concerning the biopsy utility

A pioneer work done by Theodossi et al.[53] observed a significant agreement between doctors on the liver biopsy decision. All the kappa concordance tests were significant but far from perfection (kappa = 1.00) on the following items: decision to perform biopsy (kappa = 0.42), biopsy necessary (kappa = 0.41), biopsy wanted and considered safe (kappa = 0.52), findings likely to be helpful but potential risk outweighs benefit (kappa = 0.36), and liver biopsy necessary despite the risks (kappa = 0.38). Hepatologists already had significantly heterogeneous opinions concerning the appropriateness of liver biopsy.

In a French survey 50% of HCV patients refused liver biopsy.[54]

Table 34.8 Uncontrolled observations of adverse events and mortality associated with liver biopsy.

Publication year	First author	Number of patients	Type of biopsy	Design	Adverse events definition	Severe adverse events N (per thousand, 95% CI)	Mortality N (per thousand, 95% CI)
1979	Gayral	2 346	Laparoscopy, percutaneous surgery	Retrospective	Bleeding	11 (4.7; 2.3–8.4)	4 (1.7; 0.5–4.4)
1982	Lebrec	932	Transvenous	Retrospective	Bleeding	1 (1.1; 0.3–6.0)	1 (1.1; 0.3–6.0)
1986	Piccinino	68 276	Intercostal	Retrospective	Bleeding, pneumothorax, biliary peritonitis	137 (2.0; 1.7–2.4)	5 (0.07; 0.02–0.017)
1990	McGill	9 212	Percutaneous	Retrospective	Bleeding	22 (2.4; 1.5–3.6)	10 (1.1; 0.5–2.0)
1992	Maharaj	2 646	Percutaneous	Prospective	Bleeding, pneumothorax, biliary peritonitis, pain	63 (24; 18–30)	8 (3.0; 1.3–5.9)
1993	Van Thiel	12 750	Percutaneous transplant center	Retrospective	"Major complications"	26 (2.0; 1.3–3.0)	0 (0.0; 0.0–0.3)
1993	Janes	405	Percutaneous outpatients	Retrospective	Admission	13 (32; 17–54)	0 (0.0; 0.0–9.1)
1995	Gilmore	1 500	Percutaneous	Retrospective	Bleeding	26 (17; 11–25)	5 (3.3; 1.1–7.8)
1998	Vivas	378	Percutaneous	Prospective	Admissions and bleeding	7 (19; 7–38)	0 (0.0; 0.0–9.7)
	Total	**98 445**				**306 (3.1; 2.8–3.5)**	**33 (0.3; 0.2–0.5)**

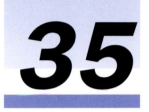

Advantage and limits of biochemical markers

Historical experience

Since the introduction of biochemical tests and ultrasound, physicians have tried to replace liver biopsy by noninvasive markers.[53] The milestones in this research were the discovery of transaminases[55] and hepatitis B virus antigen[56] and the development of the hepatitis C virus antibody assay[57] (Table 35.1).

Table 35.1 Milestones in biological markers reducing the need of liver biopsy for chronic viral hepatitis.

1936	Discovery of the transaminases by Bronstein
1965	Discovery of Australian antigen by Blumberg
1989	Discovery of HCV virus antibody by Houghton

Overview of biochemical markers

A recent overview analyzed 66 studies of tests predicting biopsy findings.[13] Most of the studies used a cross-sectional or diagnostic test design, but a few studies used a prospective cohort design. In only three studies was a first set of patients used to develop a statistical model predicting fibrosis, and the results were validated in an independent second set of patients[58–60] (Table 35.2).

Serum aminotransferases

Serum alanine aminotransferase (ALT) was the most commonly investigated marker, with sensitivity ranging from

Table 35.2 Diagnostic value of biochemical markers for fibrosis staging in patients with chronic hepatitis C.

First author	Number	Methodology	Marker	Stage	AUROC
Imbert-Bismut, 2001	205	Prospective	FibroTest	F2F3F4	0.84
	134	Prospective validation	FibroTest	F2F3F4	0.87
Poynard, 2001	461	Retrospective RCT	FibroTest	F3F4	0.74*
			Hyaluronan	F3F4	0.65
Poynard, 2002	352	Retrospective RCT	FibroTest	F2F3F4	0.73
	352	Retrospective RCT	FibroTest	F2F3F4	0.77
Myers, 2002	534	Prospective	FibroTest	F2F3F4	0.79
			FibroTest	F3F4	0.88
			FibroTest	F4	0.90
Rossi, 2003	125	Prospective	FibroTest	F2F3F4	0.74
Myers, 2003	130	Retrospective VIH	FibroTest	F2F3F4	0.86
Myers, 2002	1570	Retrospective	FibroTest	F2F3F4	0.78
			FibroTest	F4	0.87
			FibroTest	F3F4	0.83
			FibroTest	F1	0.88
			FibroTest	F0	0.82
Forns, 2002	351	Prospective	Forns Index	F2F3F4	0.86
	125	Prospective validation	Forns Index	F2F3F4	0.81
Thabut, 2003	249	Retrospective	FibroTest	F2F3F4	0.84**
			Forns Index	F2F3F4	0.78
Le Calvez 2004	323	Retrospective	FibroTest	F2F3F4	0.83†
			APRI Index	F2F3F4	0.74
Callewaert 2004	82	Prospective	FibroTest	F3F4	0.89
			GlycocirrhoTest	F3F4	0.87
Guechot, 1996	176	Prospective	Hyaluronan	F3F4	0.86***
			P-III-P	F3F4	0.69
Lo Iacono, 1998	52	Retrospective	P-III-P	F3F4	0.73
Walsh, 1999	33	Prospective	P-III-P CIS	F3F4	0.76
			P-III-P Orion	F3F4	0.67
Walsh, 2000	37	Prospective	Collagen IV	F3F4	0.83
			Laminin	F3F4	0.82

AUROC: area under the receiver operating characteristics curve.
P-III-P: amino-terminal peptide of type III procollagen.
*FibroTest AUROC was significantly higher than Hyaluronan AUROC.
**FibroTest AUROC was significantly higher than Forns Index AUROC.
***Hyaluronan AUROC was significantly greater than P-III-P AUROC.
†FibroTest AUROC was significantly greater than APRI AUROC.

61% to 71%. The diagnostic value was lower than for the combination of markers,[60] for diagnosis of both cirrhosis and bridging fibrosis. Studies were relatively consistent in showing that serum aminotransferases have only a modest value in predicting fibrosis on liver biopsy. The fibrosis index permits the diagnosis of fibrosis among patients with normal transaminases.[60]

Extracellular matrix tests

Among the extracellular matrix tests, hyaluronic acid (Hyaluronan) correlated best with fibrosis stage overall, but this has been demonstrated for extensive fibrosis without study on a high number of patients with moderate fibrosis[13] (Table 35.2). The hyaluronic acid area under the receiver characteristics curve (AUROC) for F3F4 fibrosis stages ranged from 0.65 to 0.86.[61,62] The type III collagen peptides AUROC for F3F4 fibrosis stages ranged from 0.67 to 0.76.[61,63,64] In one very small sample size study, the laminin AUROC was 0.82, and the collagen IV AUROC was 0.83.[65] Markers of extracellular matrix degradation, such as tissue inhibitor of metalloproteinase-1-4, were also associated with fibrosis as single markers, but generally were less predictive than hyaluronic acid.[13]

Cytokines and cytokine receptors

Several cytokines and cytokine receptors were investigated, including the tumor necrosis factors (TNF), TNF-R55, TNF-R75, and TNF-alfa, as well as serum interleukin-10, and interleukin (IL)-2 receptors. Except for TNF-alfa, the cytokine and cytokine receptors were associated with fibrosis, but were less predictive than markers of extracellular matrix or panel tests. In contrast, TNF-alfa was associated with hepatic inflammation, but not with fibrosis.[13,58]

Other isolated tests

Other tests were investigated, including glutathione, alfa-fetoprotein, prothrombin time, pseudocholinesterase, manganese superoxide dismutase, beta-*N*-galactosidase, alfa 2-macroglobin, beta-globulin, albumin, glutamyl transpeptidase, bilirubin, lactate dehydrogenase, aspartate aminotransferase (AST), alkaline phosphatase, white blood cell count, creatinine, total bile acids, and immunoglobulin G. These markers were less useful as a group than the other markers discussed.[13] The platelet count, an indicator of portal hypertension, is also a predictor of cirrhosis, both in isolation and in studies using panels of markers.[13,56,65]

Other test panels

Panels of markers have the greatest value in predicting the absence or no more than minimal fibrosis on biopsy and in predicting the presence of cirrhosis on biopsy.[13]

Five studies[56–58,60,64] used large panels of markers and achieved the greatest predictive values, with sensitivities ranging from 50% to 82%, and specificities ranging from 35% to 80%. A panel of matrix metalloprotein-2, 7S type IV collagen, and hyaluronic acid predicted no fibrosis/minimal fibrosis, with a sensitivity of 68% and specificity of 73%.[64] Up to 94% of cirrhotic patients could be correctly identified by multivariate models. A multivariate model using age and platelets, moderate to severe inflammation and/or bridging fibrosis or cirrhosis could be identified with a specificity of 95% and sensitivity of 52%.[56] An index combining age, platelets, gamma-glutamyl transpeptidase (GGT) and cholesterol showed good diagnostic value, with an AUROC at 0.81.[66] One weakness of this index is the variability of serum cholesterol according to steatosis, particularly in patients infected by HCV genotype 3.[67]

An index combining AST and platelets showed good diagnostic value with an AUROC at 0.83.[68,69] One weakness is the prevalence of patients with normal transaminases and extensive fibrosis.[69]

FibroTest and ActiTest

Since the Gebo et al. review,[13] a total of 16 studies have been published on two combinations of biochemical markers,[58,60,69,72–81] including patients coinfected with HCV and HIV.[73]

One combination is called the fibrosis index (FibroTest), combining the following five markers: α_2-macroglobulin, haptoglobin, GGT, total bilirubin, and apolipoprotein A1.[58] A positive correlation between α_2-macroglobulin and fibrosis has been reported in alcoholic liver disease and chronic hepatitis C and B. Since α_2-macroglobulin is a protease inhibitor expressed by activated hepatic stellate cells, increased synthesis may enhance fibrosis by inhibiting the catabolism of extracellular matrix proteins. Apolipoprotein A1 is reduced in patients with advanced fibrosis. In vitro studies and biopsies showing deposition on fibrous septa implicate binding of this protein within the extracellular matrix. The negative association between haptoglobulin and fibrosis may be due to its association with TGF-β1, a profibrogenic cytokine.[58]

The second combination is called the activity index (ActiTest). It combined the same five markers plus ALT and has a high predictive value for the diagnosis of significant necroinflammatory, histologic activity.

FibroTest-ActiTest is on the US market with the name HCU-FibroSure™.

A summary of the diagnostic value of the FibroTest in patients with chronic hepatitis C is shown in Table 35.2. Similar diagnostic values have been observed in 249 patients with chronic hepatitis B, for the diagnosis of both moderate and extensive fibrosis (FibroTest AUROC = 0.78) and for moderate or severe activity (ActiTest AUROC = 0.82). FibroTest scores of ≤0.20 and >0.80 had negative and positive predictive values of 92%, respectively.

The advantages of the FibroTest and ActiTest are to give two quantitative and continuous estimates of both fibrosis and activity, with a conversion to the classical fibrosis stage and activity grades of the METAVIR scoring system (Table 35.3 and Figure 35.1).

Table 35.3 Conversion between FibroTest values and fibrosis stages and between ActiTest values and activity grades.

FibroTest	Estimate of fibrosis stage	ActiTest	Estimate of activity grade
0.75–1.00	F4		
0.73–0.74	F3–F4	0.62–1.00	A3
0.59–0.72	F3	0.61–0.61	A2–A3
0.49–0.58	F2	0.53–0.60	A2
0.32–0.48	F1–F2	0.37–0.52	A1–A2
0.28–0.31	F1	0.30–0.36	A1
0.22–0.27	F0–F1	0.18–0.29	A0–A1
0.00–0.21	F0	0.00–0.17	A0

F0: no fibrosis; F1: portal fibrosis; F2: little bridging; F3: much bridging; F4: cirrhosis; A0: no activity; A1: minimal activity; A2: moderate activity; A3: severe activity.

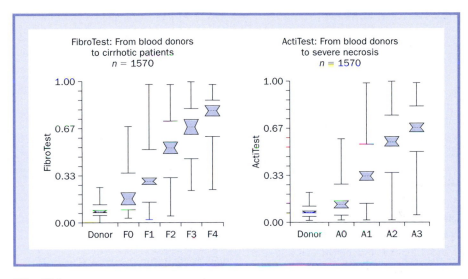

Figure 35.1
Conversion between FibroTest values and fibrosis stages and between ActiTest values and activity grades.

Table 35.4 Summary of advantages and limits of liver biopsy and biochemical markers.

	Liver biopsy	Biochemical markers
History	Classical standard	New tests or panel tests
Disease diagnosis	Fibrosis, activity, steatosis, iron	Fibrosis, activity (transaminases, ActiTest)
Estimate	Semiquantitative	Quantitative and continuous
False negative	Regeneration nodule	Acute inflammation
False positive	Subcapsular biopsy	Hemolysis, Gilbert's disease, acute hepatitis, extrahepatic cholestasis, acute inflammation
Adverse events	3 deaths out of 10 000 3 severe adverse events out of 1000 30 painful out of 100	None
Sampling error	33% discordance in fibrosis staging 24% discordance in activity grading	None
Observer error	Fibrosis stage discordance (20%) Activity grade discordance (40%)	Coefficient variation lower than 5%
Minimal requirements	At least 25 mm size More than 5 portal tracts	Standardized assays, kits and analyzers
Hospitalization	6–24 h	None
Contraindications	Coagulation disorder, risk of respiratory insufficiency	None
Cost	US$1032 for uncomplicated biopsy; US$2745 for complicated biopsy	90–300 euro for FibroTest–ActiTest–FibroSure

The limitations of the FibroTest and ActiTest are false-positive findings due to hemolysis (decrease of haptoglobin and increase of nonconjugated bilirubin), to Gilbert's disease (increase in non-conjugated bilirubin) and to extrahepatic cholestasis (increase in total bilirubin and GGT). In acute inflammation, false positives are possible (increase in α2 macroglobulin) as well as false negative (increase in haptoglobin).

Comparison between biochemical markers

For the prediction of moderate fibrosis stage, the FibroTest diagnostic value was greater than several isolated markers, including transaminases,[58] hyaluronic acid,[60] historical features,[70] prothrombin time,[72] age and platelet index,[72] the index combining GGT, age, platelets and cholesterol,[69] and the APRI index.[71] Hyaluronic acid was superior to P-III-P for the diagnosis of extensive fibrosis.[59]

The future of proteomics

Serum protein profiling already achieved promising predictive values for the diagnosis of significant fibrosis in preliminary study.[83] Profiles of serum protein N-glycans have recently demonstrated good diagnostic value for the diagnosis of cirrhosis, with 79% sensitivity and 86% specificity. The AUROC (0.87) was, however, similar to that of FibroTest (0.89).[84]

References

1. Von Frerichs. *Über den Diabetes*. Berlin: Hirschwald, 1884.

2. Schupfer F. De la possibilité de faire "intra vitam" un diagnostic précis des maladies du foie et de la rate. *Semin Med* 1907; **27**: 229–30.

3. Huard P. La ponction biopsie du foie et son utilité dans le diagnostic des affections hépatiques. *Ann Anat Pathol* 1935; **12**: 1118–24.

4. Menghini G. One-second needle biopsy of the liver. *Gastroenterology* 1958; **35**: 190–9.

5. Perrillo RP. The role of liver biopsy in hepatitis C. *Hepatology* 1997; **26**: 57S–61S.

6. EASL International Consensus Conference on Hepatitis C. Consensus statement. *J Hepatol* 1999; **30**: 956–61.

7. Consensus conference treatment of hepatitis C. Guidelines. *Gastroenterol Clin Biol* 2002; **2**: B312–20.

8. National Institutes of Health Consensus Development Conference Statement. Management of hepatitis C: 2002. *Hepatology* 2002; **36**: S35–46.

9. Lok AS, Heathcote EJ, Hoofnagle JH. Management of hepatitis B: 2000—summary of a workshop. *Gastroenterology* 2001; **120**: 1828–53.

10. Valla D. EASL Jury. EASL international consensus conference on hepatitis B. *J Hepatol* 2003; **38**: 533–40.

11. Bravo AA, Sheth SG, Chopra S. Liver biopsy. *N Engl J Med* 2001; **344**: 495–500.

12. Dienstag JL. The role of liver biopsy in chronic hepatitis C. *Hepatology* 2002; **36**: S152–60.

13. Gebo KA, Herlong HF, Torbenson MS, et al. Role of liver biopsy in management of chronic hepatitis C: A systematic review. *Hepatology* 2002; **36**: S161–72.

14. Poynard T, Lebrec D. The inconvenience of investigations used in hepatology: patients' and hepatologists' opinions. *Liver* 1982; **2**: 369–75.

15. Poynard T, Ratziu V, Bedossa P. Appropriateness of liver biopsy. *Can J Gastroenterol* 2000; **14**: 543–8.

16. Knodell KG, Ishak KG, Black WC, et al. Formulation and application of a numerical scoring system for assessing histological activity in asymptomatic chronic active hepatitis. *Hepatology* 1981; **1**: 431–5.

17. Ludwig J. The nomenclature of chronic active hepatitis: An obituary. *Gastroenterology* 1993; **105**: 274–8.

18. Bedossa P, Poynard T. The METAVIR cooperative group. Inter- and intra-observer variation in the assessment of liver biopsy of chronic hepatitis C. *Hepatology* 1994; **20**(1): 15–20.

19. Ishak K, Baptista A, Bianchi L, et al. Histological grading and staging of chronic hepatitis. *J Hepatol* 1995; **22**: 696–9.

20. Bedossa P, Poynard T. An algorithm for the grading of activity in chronic hepatitis C. METAVIR Cooperative Study Group. *Hepatology* 1996; **24**: 289–93.

21. Poynard T, Bedossa P, Opolon P. Natural history of liver fibrosis progression in patients with chronic hepatitis C. The OBSVIRC, METAVIR, CLINIVIR, and DOSVIRC groups. *Lancet* 1997; **349**: 825–32.

22. Poynard T, Ratziu V, Benmanov Y, et al. Fibrosis in patients with chronic hepatitis C: Detection and significance. *Semin Liver Dis* 2000; **20**: 47–55.

23. Deuffic-Burban S, Poynard T, Valleron AJ. Quantification of fibrosis progression in patients with chronic hepatitis C using a Markov model. *J Viral Hepat* 2002; **9**: 114–22.

24. Poynard T, Mathurin P, Lai CL, et al. A comparison of fibrosis progression in chronic liver diseases. *J Hepatol* 2003; **38**: 257–65.

25. Crawford AR, Lin XZ, Crawford JM. The normal adult human liver biopsy: A quantitative reference standard. *Hepatology* 1998; **28**: 323–31.

26. Urena MA, Ruiz-Delgado FC, Gonzalez EM, et al. Assessing risk of the use of livers with macro and microsteatosis in a liver transplant program. *Transplant Proc* 1998; **30**: 3288–91.

27. Klatskin G, Conn HO. *Histopathology of the Liver*. New York: Oxford University Press, 1993.

28. Bedossa P, Dargare D, Paradis V. Sampling variability of liver fibrosis in chronic hepatitis C. *Hepatology* 2003; **38**: 1449–57.

29. Soloway RD, Baggenstoss AH, Schoenfield LJ, Summerskill WH. Observer error and sampling variability tested in evaluation of hepatitis and cirrhosis by liver biopsy. *Am J Dig Dis* 1971; **16**: 1082–6.

30. Labayle D, Chaput JC, Albuisson F, et al. Analyse histologique comparative des biopsies du lobe droit et du lobe gauche dans les lésions alcooliques du foie. *Gastroenterol Clin Biol* 1979; **3**: 235–40.

31. Abdi W, Millan JC, Mezey E. Sampling variability on percutaneous liver biopsy. *Arch Intern Med* 1979; **139**: 667–9.

32. Schlichting P, Holund B, Poulsen H. Liver biopsy in chronic aggressive hepatitis. Diagnostic reproducibility in relation to size of specimen. *Scand J Gastroenterol* 1983; **18**: 27–32.

33. Maharaj B, Maharaj RJ, Leary WP, et al. Sampling variability and its influence on the diagnostic yield of percutaneous needle biopsy of the liver. *Lancet* 1986; **1**: 523–5.

34. Regev A, Berho M, Jeffers LJ, et al. Sampling error and intraobserver variation in liver biopsy in patients with chronic HCV infection. *Am J Gastroenterol* 2002; **97**: 2614–18.

35. Christoffersen P, Poulsen H, Skeie E. Focal liver necrosis accompanied by infiltration of granulocytes arising during operation. *Acta Hepato-Splenologica* 1970; **17**: 240–5.

36. Herrerias JM, Company FP, Osorio M, Garrido M. Discrepancias entre el diagnostico laparoscopico e histologico en la cirrhosis

hepatica. *Rev Esp Enferm Ap Dig* 1974; **42:** 709–14.

37. Poniachik J, Bernstein DE, Reddy KR, et al. The role of laparoscopy in the diagnosis of cirrhosis. *Gastrointest Endosc* 1996; **43:** 568–71.

38. Pagliaro L, Rinaldi F, Craxi A, et al. Percutaneous blind biopsy versus laparoscopy with guided biopsy in diagnosis of cirrhosis. A prospective, randomized trial. *Dig Dis Sci* 1983; **28:** 39–43.

39. Westin J, Lagging LM, Wejstal R, Norkrans G, Dhillon AP. Interobserver study of liver histopathology using the Ishak score in patients with chronic hepatitis C virus infection. *Liver* 1999; **19:** 183–7.

40. Gronbaek K, Christensen PB, Hamilton-Dutoit S, et al. Interobserver variation in interpretation of serial liver biopsies from patients with chronic hepatitis C. *J Viral Hepat* 2002; **9:** 443–9.

41. Theodossi A, Skene AM, Portmann B. Observer variation in assessment of liver biopsies including analysis by kappa statistics. *Gastroenterology* 1980; **79:** 232–41.

42. Petz D, Klauck S, Rohl FW, et al. Feasibility of histological grading and staging of chronic viral hepatitis using specimens obtained by thin-needle biopsy. *Virchows Arch* 2003; **442:** 238–44.

43. Gayral F, Potier M, Salmon R, Labayle D, Larrieu H. Vascular complications of needle biopsy of the liver. *J Chir (Paris)* 1979; **116:** 261–4.

44. Lebrec D, Goldfarb G, Degott C, Rueff B, Benhamou JP. Transvenous liver biopsy: An experience based on 1000 hepatic tissue samplings with this procedure. *Gastroenterology* 1982; **83:** 338–40.

45. Piccinino F, Sagnelli E, Pasquale G, Giusti G. Complications following percutaneous liver biopsy. A multicentre retrospective study on 68,276 biopsies. *J Hepatol* 1986; **2:** 165–73.

46. McGill DB, Rakela J, Zinsmeister AR, Ott BJ. A 21-year experience with major

hemorrhage after percutaneous liver biopsy. *Gastroenterology* 1990; **99:** 1396–400.

47. Maharaj B, Bhoora IG. Complications associated with percutaneous needle biopsy of the liver when one, two or three specimens are taken. *Postgrad Med J* 1992; **68:** 964–7.

48. Van Thiel DH, Gavaler JS, Wright H, Tzakis A. Liver biopsy. Its safety and complications as seen at a liver transplant center. *Transplantation* 1993; **55:** 1087–90.

49. Janes CH, Lindor KD. Outcome of patients hospitalized for complications after outpatient liver biopsy. *Ann Intern Med* 1993; **118:** 96–8.

50. Gilmore IT, Burroughs A, Murray-Lyon IM, et al. Indications, methods, and outcomes of percutaneous liver biopsy in England and Wales: An audit by the British Society of Gastroenterology and the Royal College of Physicians of London. *Gut* 1995; **36:** 437–41.

51. Vivas S, Palacio MA, Rodriguez M, et al. Ambulatory liver biopsy: Complications and evolution in 264 cases. *Rev Esp Enferm Dig* 1998; **90:** 175–82.

52. Wong JB, Koff RS. Watchful waiting with periodic liver biopsy versus immediate empirical therapy for histologically mild chronic hepatitis C. A cost-effectiveness analysis. *Ann Intern Med* 2000; **133:** 665–75.

53. Theodossi A, Spiegelhalter D, Portmann B, Eddleston AL, Williams R. The value of clinical, biochemical, ultrasound and liver biopsy data in assessing patients with liver disease. *Liver* 1983; **3:** 315–26.

54. Bonny C, Rayssiguier R, Ughetto S, et al. Medical practices and expectations of general practitioners in relation to hepatitis C virus infection in the Auvergne region. *Gastroenterol Clin Biol* 2003; **27:** 1021–5.

55. Cooper AJ, Meister A. An appreciation of Professor Alexander E. Braunstein. The discovery and scope of enzymatic transamination. *Biochimie* 1989; **71:** 387–404.

56. Alter HJ, Blumberg BS. Further studies on a

"new" human isoprecipitin system (Australia antigen). *Blood* 1966; **27**: 297–309.

57.   Kuo G, Choo QL, Alter HJ, et al. An assay for circulating antibodies to a major etiologic virus of human non-A, non-B hepatitis. *Science* 1989; **244**: 362–4.

58.   Poynard T, Bedossa P. Age and platelet count: A simple index for predicting the presence of histological lesions in patients with antibodies to hepatitis C virus. METAVIR and CLINIVIR Cooperative Study Groups. *J Viral Hepat* 1997; **4**: 199–208.

59.   Fortunato G, Castaldo G, Oriani G, et al. Multivariate discriminant function based on six biochemical markers in blood can predict the cirrhotic evolution of chronic hepatitis. *Clin Chem* 2001; **47**: 1696–1700.

60.   Imbert-Bismut F, Ratziu V, Pieroni L, et al. Biochemical markers of liver fibrosis in patients with hepatitis C virus infection: A prospective study. *Lancet* 2001; **357**: 1069–75.

61.   Guechot J, Laudat A, Loria A, et al. Diagnostic accuracy of hyaluronan and type III procollagen amino-terminal peptide serum assays as markers of liver fibrosis in chronic viral hepatitis C evaluated by ROC curve analysis. *Clin Chem* 1996; **42**: 558–63.

62.   Poynard T, Imbert-Bismut F, Ratziu V, et al. Biochemical markers of liver fibrosis in patients infected by hepatitis C virus: Longitudinal validation in a randomized trial. *J Viral Hepat* 2002; **9**: 128–33.

63.   Lo Iacono O, Garcia-Monzon C, Almasio P, et al. Soluble adhesion molecules correlate with liver inflammation and fibrosis in chronic hepatitis C treated with interferon-alpha. *Aliment Pharmacol Ther* 1998; **12**: 1091–9.

64.   Walsh KM, Fletcher A, MacSween RN, Morris AJ. Comparison of assays for N-amino terminal propeptide of type III procollagen in chronic hepatitis C by using receiver operating characteristic analysis. *Eur J Gastroenterol Hepatol* 1999; **1**: 827–31.

65.   Walsh KM, Fletcher A, MacSween RN,

Morris AJ. Basement membrane peptides as markers of liver disease in chronic hepatitis C. *J Hepatol* 2000; **32**: 325–30.

66.   Murawaki Y, Ikuta Y, Okamoto K, Koda M, Kawasaki H. Diagnostic value of serum markers of connective tissue turnover for predicting histological staging and grading in patients with chronic hepatitis C. *J Gastroenterol* 2001; **36**: 399–406.

67.   Ono E, Shiratori Y, Okudaira T, et al. Platelet count reflects stage of chronic hepatitis C. *Hepatol Res* 1999; **15**: 192–200.

68.   Forns X, Ampurdanes S, Llovet JM, et al. Identification of chronic hepatitis C patients without hepatic fibrosis by a simple predictive model. *Hepatology* 2002; **36**: 986–92.

69.   Thabut D, Simon M, Myers RP, et al. Noninvasive prediction of fibrosis in patients with chronic hepatitis C [Letter]. *Hepatology* 2003; **37**: 1220–1.

70.   Wai CT, Greenson JK, Fontana RJ, et al. A simple non invasive index can predict both significant fibrosis and cirrhosis in patients with chronic hepatitis C. *Hepatology* 2003; **38**: 518–26

71.   Le Calvez S, Thabut D, Messous D, et al. FibroTest has higher predictive values than APRI for fibrosis diagnosis in patients with chronic hepatitis C. *Hepatology* 2004; **39**: 862–3.

72.   Myers RP, Ratziu V, Charlotte F, Imbert-Bismut F, Poynard T. Biochemical markers of liver fibrosis: A comparison with historical features in patients with chronic hepatitis C. *Am J Gastroenterol* 2002; **97**: 2419–25.

73.   Halfon P, Imbert-Bismut F, Messous D, et al. A prospective assessment of the inter-laboratory variability of biochemical markers of fibrosis (FibroTest) and activity (ActiTest) in patients with chronic liver disease. *Comp Hepatol* 2002; **2**: 3–6.

74.   Myers RP, de Torres M, Imbert-Bismut F, et al. Biochemical markers of fibrosis in patients with chronic hepatitis C: A comparison with prothrombin time, platelet count and the age-platelet index. *Dig Dis Sci* 2003; **48**: 146–53.

75. Myers RP, Benhamou Y, Imbert-Bismut F, et al. Serum biochemical markers accurately predict liver fibrosis in HIV and hepatitis C virus-coinfected patients. *AIDS* 2003; **17**: 721–5.

76. Myers RP, Messous D, Thabut D, et al. Life is possible without biopsy in patients with chronic hepatitis C: Validation of biochemical markers of liver fibrosis and activity in 1570 patients and blood donors [Abstract]. *Hepatology* 2002; **36**: 351A.

77. Poynard T, McHutchison J, Manns M, Myers RP, Albrecht J. Biochemical surrogate markers of liver fibrosis and activity in a randomized trial of peginterferon alfa-2b and ribavirin. *Hepatology* 2003; **38**: 481–92.

78. Myers RP, Messous D, Thabut D, et al. The prediction of fibrosis with serum biochemical markers in patients with chronic hepatitis C: Prospective validation in 534 patients [Abstract]. *Hepatology* 2002; **36**: 351A.

79. Adams L, Rossi E, DeBoer B, et al. Use of FibroTest to predict liver fibrosis in hepatitis C: A replacement for liver biopsy? [Abstract]. *Gastroenterology* 2002; **122**: 1615A.

80. Rossi E, Adams L, Prins A, et al. Validation of the FibroTest biochemical markers score in assessing liver fibrosis in hepatitis C patients. *Clin Chem* 2003; **49**: 450–4.

81. Poynard T, Imbert-Bismut F, Ratziu V, et al. FibroTest even better than liver biopsy? *Clin Chem* 2003. Electronic letter www.clinchem.org/cgi/eletters/49/3/450. Response: 21 March 2003.

82. Myers R, Tainturier MH, Ratziu V, et al. Prediction of liver histological lesions with biochemical markers in patients with chronic hepatitis B. *J Hepatol* 2003; **39**: 222–30.

83. Paradis V, Bonvoust F, Ratziu V, Dargere D, Poynard T, Belossa P. Serum protein profiling of patients with chronic hepatitis C by SELDITOF Protein chip: A new approach to surrogate markers of liver fibrosis. *Hepatology* 2002; **36**: 352A.

84. Callewaert N, Van Vlierberghe H, Van Hecke A, Laroy W, Delanghe J, Conteras R. Non invasive diagnosis of liver cirrhosis using DNA sequencer-based total serum protein glycomics. *Nature Med* 2004; **10**: 429–34.

Index